Advances in Body Composition Assessment

Current Issues in Exercise Science

Monograph Number 3

Timothy G. Lohman, PhD
University of Arizona

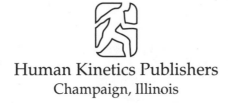

Human Kinetics Publishers
Champaign, Illinois

Library of Congress Cataloging-in-Publication Data

Lohman, Timothy G. 1940-
  Advances in body composition assessment / Timothy G. Lohman.
      p.   cm. -- (Current issues in exercise science ; monograph no.
  3)
  Includes bibliographical references and index.
  ISBN 0-87322-327-6
  1. Body composition.   I. Title.   II. Series.
  [DNLM: 1. Anthropometry--methods. 2. Body Composition. QU 100
  L833a]
  QP88.L65   1992
  612--dc20
  DNLM/DLC
  for Library of Congress   92-1476
                                                                              CIP

ISBN: 0-87322-327-6
ISSN: 1055-1352

Managing Editor: Julia Anderson
Assistant Editor: Moyra Knight
Copyeditor: Wendy Nelson
Proofreader: Laurie McGee
Indexer: Theresa Schaefer
Production Director: Ernie Noa
Typesetting and Text Layout: Angela K. Snyder
Text Design: Keith Blomberg
Cover Design: Hunter Graphics
Interior Art: Gretchen Walters
Printer: United Graphics

Printed in the United States of America

10 9 8 7 6 5 4 3 2 1

Human Kinetics Publishers
Box 5076, Champaign, IL 61825-5076
1-800-747-4457

Canada Office:
Human Kinetics Publishers, Inc.
P.O. Box 2503, Windsor, ON N8Y 4S2
1-800-465-7301 (in Canada only)

Europe Office
Human Kinetics Publishers (Europe) Ltd.
P.O. Box IW14
Leeds LS16 6TR
England
0532-781708

To J. Fleur Lohman, who has supported and encouraged me in both my professional and personal development over the past 32 years.

Contents

Preface

My introduction to the field of body composition began in 1962 as I was completing my undergraduate training in agricultural science at the University of Illinois. At that time the animal science department was acquiring a whole-body liquid scintillation counter to assess body composition in farm animals and humans by measuring naturally occurring potassium-40. Over the next 5 years as a graduate research student, I learned much about the development and validation of a new body composition method, and I began to grow in appreciation for the science and methodology of body composition assessment. The challenge of developing indirect methods for better estimation of lean, bone, and fat and the application of these methods to many fields of study continued to provide for me an exciting and rewarding research discipline over the next 30 years. The perspective of this field that I've gained over the years is the basis for this monograph.

In its goals and scope, this monograph differs from many of the excellent review articles that have outlined the theory, advantages, and limitations of the various approaches to body composition assessment. In this monograph, I refer to many important works that chronicle advances in the field, including Hines (1991), Lukaski (1987), the Ross Conference on Body Composition Assessment in Youth and Adults (Roche, 1985), the original work of Siri (1961), and many articles in the *Annals of the New York Academy of Sciences* (e.g., Brozek, Grande, Anderson, & Kemp, 1963), especially the article on the three-component model by Anderson (1963). For a comprehensive understanding of the many aspects of body composition measurement, you may want to review G.B. Forbes's 1987 publication, *Human Body Composition*, and *Evaluation and Regulation of Body Build and Composition* by A.R. Behnke and J.H. Wilmore (1974).

My goal in writing this monograph is to explore some of the issues, concepts, and controversies in the context of advances in the study of body composition. This is intended to give both researchers and students attracted to the field an overview of some of the critical areas and questions under exploration, many of which are not yet resolved. Traditional approaches in body composition assessment include using height and weight as indices of obesity; using the two-component system of estimating fat and fat-free body mass for describing body composition changes associated with growth and development, exercise, dietary restriction, and aging, as well as for validating new methods; and using body mass index or waist-to-hip ratio for the estimation of fat distribution. I intend to make the need to go beyond such approaches evident throughout this monograph. Developing better approaches to body composition assessment will lead to a better understanding of growth and development, aging and disease, and the effects of exercise and dietary restriction on body composition, as well as provide sound criteria for validating new methods of assessment.

From a scientific and technological perspective, new methods of estimating body composition, such as whole-body electrical impedance, total body electrical conductivity, and dual energy X-ray absorptiometry offer alternative methodologies for body composition measurement in various settings in addition to the traditional methods of densitometry, hydrometry, and anthropometry. Multicomponent models are also receiving considerable attention from leading researchers. In chapters 1 through 4, I deal with some of the issues related to these methodological advances.

A crucial question in the field relates to the relative risk of total body fatness versus fat distribution in relation to diabetes, hypertension, blood lipids, and coronary heart disease. In chapter 5, I address the conceptual issues to enable better assessment of fat distribution to help resolve this critical question.

In chapter 6, I explore the estimation of body composition in children and the elderly and the problems of using the two-component system, and I examine revised estimates of the prevalence of obesity in children and youth in chapter 7. In chapter 8, I explore evidence examining the tracking of body composition from infancy to adulthood. In chapter 9, I present implications for youth fitness, based on the information in chapters 6 to 8. I examine the application of body composition assessment to estimates of minimal weight in the athletic population in chapter 10, emphasizing the high school wrestling population as a model cross-validation research study to develop a generalized skinfold equation in this population. In the final chapter I highlight some of the recent advances in assessement methods, such as multifrequency, bioelectric impedance, infrared reactance, and total body electrical conductivity, and look at the role of industry in the development of new methodologies.

Acknowledgments

I want to express my appreciation for many interchanges I have had, in writing this book, with colleagues and mentors, each of whom has contributed to the ideas and substance of this book: Joy Bunt, Dick Boileau, Claude Bouchard, Elsworth Buskirk, Connie Christ, Scott Going, Linda Houtkooper, Tony Jackson, Joe Kastelic, Bob Malina, Tod Norton, Mike Pollock, Arie Selinger, Wayne Sinning, Mary Slaughter, Fred Roby, Alex Roche, Bob Twardock, Charles Tipton, and Jack Wilmore; to those teachers whom I have met primarily through their ideas and works, I want to acknowledge Ernest Anderson, Albert Behnke, Joseph Brozek, Gilbert Forbes, and William Siri.

Chapter 1

Basic Concepts in Body Composition Assessment

Any student of body composition must master terminology and the concepts of validation scales for assessing the effectiveness of new methods, new methods to assess regional as well as total body composition, and the need for population-specific equations. Lack of understanding these concepts has hindered the development of the field.

I begin this chapter with my general perspective on the field of body composition assessment, briefly outlining recent advances in the field and remaining areas of concern. Basic concepts such as fat-free body mass and lean body mass are presented and various terms are defined for the purposes of this book. The validation of new methods of body composition assessment, including the two-component model, are examined. The need for new reference methods is also explored, highlighting regional estimates of body composition and population-specific body composition equations. The chapter's contents provide a useful frame of reference for the remaining chapters of the book.

The Field of Body Composition Assessment

The field of body composition assessment is developing rapidly on several fronts. Some of the major areas are the estimation of the fat and fat-free body composition of the body and sources of variation in that composition associated with growth and senescence, physical activity, and specific exercise training programs, along with ethnic and gender patterns of fat distribution and differential development of the musculoskeletal system.

The relation of body composition to health is another front on which much research is being conducted. Methodological developments applied to large-scale epidemiological studies are needed to better define the health issues related to fatness versus fat distribution. The use of body mass index has dominated this field in the past, confounding fat, muscle, and bone content in relation to health risk. The association of body composition with risk of diabetes, hypertension, blood lipid and lipoprotein profile, and coronary heart disease needs additional attention. Traditional measures of anthropometry and height and weight have been expanded to examine fat distribution (e.g., waist-to-hip ratio and extremity-to-trunk skinfolds with the hypothesis that abdominal fat and upper body trunkal fat are more closely tied to health risk than any other fat depots.

The application of established methodologies of body composition in large populations is another front where continued research is needed. In the 1960s in the National Health Examination Survey, in the 1970s in the NHANES I and II, and in the 1980s in the National Children's Youth Fitness Study (NCYFS) height, weight, and three to five skinfolds have been utilized to assess various national probability samples. Skinfolds have been applied to the new health-related physical fitness tests (AAHPERD Health-Related Physical Fitness Test, Fitnessgram, Fit Youth Today [Texas Fitness Test], AAHPERD Physical Best, and YMCA Youth Fitness Test) to be used throughout the nation to help youth understand more about their body composition and ways it can be modified for a healthier life. Skinfolds are being used to assess body composition in high school wrestlers to estimate minimal weight, and there is potential that a national system will be developed to help eliminate the dehydration and starvation practices in this population.

Fat-Free Body Mass Versus Lean Body Mass

Many body composition studies estimate fat-free body mass from densitometry using the Siri (1961) or Brozek et al. (1963) equation; however, they use the term *lean body mass* to denote fat-free body mass (FFB). As originally defined by Behnke (1959), lean body mass has a density less than 1.100 g/cm³ and contains a small amount of essential lipid (2% to 3%); in contrast, fat-free body mass has no lipids. I use the term *fat-free body mass* throughout this book (Table 1.1). I urge my colleagues to stay with the original definition of lean body (LBM) mass and to use *fat-free body mass* as the preferred term when body composition validation studies are conducted and the usual constants applied. Suggested constants for converting FFB to LBM and minimal weight (5% fat for men and 12% fat for women) are given in Table 1.1.

Table 1.1   Interconversion of Fat-Free Body Mass (FFB),
Lean Body Mass, and Minimal Weight

Sex	Lean body mass	Minimal weight
	Divide FFB by	
Male	.97	.95
Female	.92	.88

Validating New Methods of Assessing Body Composition

To evaluate a new method of assessing body composition, either percent fat or FFB, in kilograms, is used as the variable to be predicted from the new techniques. Errors of predicting FFB in kilograms are obtained from the prediction error, as are standard errors of estimate on variation about a linear or curvilinear regression line. Using body density as the criterion variable for the determination of FFB, I published a set of standards for judging the magnitude of the standard errors of estimate in young adult men and women (Lohman, 1991). Table 1.2 indicates that prediction errors of 2.5 kg for men and 1.8 kg for women are excellent and probably reflect errors of 1.8 kg and 1.0 kg, respectively, in the new methodology. These errors are lower than the standard error of estimate, because the criterion method itself has an error of measurement and does not allow for perfect criterion scores. Sources of these errors are carefully reviewed in chapter 2 for densitometry, but they are often ignored in the publication of prediction equations, where all the error is usually attributed to the new method in question. Until we obtain a set of reference methods in the field of body composition with an accuracy and precision of less than 1%, we will have the criterion method contributing 20% to 50% of the error between methods. In extending this table to percent-fat prediction errors, we will use a 76.5-kg man and a 60.0-kg woman with fat contents of 15% and 25%, respectively (Table 1.3). Thus, by using these two tables, we can better judge the validity of the new method in question.

Table 1.2 Fat-Free Body Mass Prediction Errors and Actual Errors (FFB, kg, Estimated From Densitometry)[a] With a Criterion Error-Free Method

Standard error of estimate, kg		Actual error using a criterion error-free method, kg		Subjective rating
Men	Women	Men	Women	
2.0-2.5	1.5-1.8	0-1.8	0-1.8	Ideal
2.5	1.8	1.8	1.0	Excellent
3.0	2.3	2.3	1.7	Very good
3.5	2.8	2.9	2.4	Good
4.0	2.8	2.9	2.4	Fairly good
4.5	3.6	4.0	3.3	Fair
>4.5	>4.0	—	—	Not recommended

Note. From "Anthropometric Assessment of Fat-Free Body Mass" by T.G. Lohman. In *Anthropometric Assessment of Nutritional Status* (p. 175) by J.H. Himes (Ed.), 1991, New York: John Wiley. Copyright © 1991 by John Wiley. Adapted by permission of Wiley-Liss, a division of John Wiley and Sons, Inc.
[a]Errors in fat-free body mass from densitometry are assumed to be 1.9 kg for men 1.5 kg for women (Lohman 1991).

Table 1.3   Percent-Fat Prediction Errors and Actual Errors (Percent Fat Estimated From Densitometry)[a] With a Criterion Error-Free Method

Standard error of estimate % Men and women	Actual error using criterion error-free methods, % Men and women	Subjective rating
2.0	0-2.0	Ideal
2.5	1.5	Excellent
3.0	2.2	Very good
3.5	2.9	Good
4.0	3.5	Fairly good
4.5	4.0	Fair
5.0	4.6	Not recomended

[a]Errors in percent fat from densitometry associated with variation in water and mineral content of the fat-free body are assumed to be 2.0%.

Two-Component Model of Validation

Many validation studies use the two-component model on a mixed sample of several populations, even though it has been established that the two-component model works well only in a specific population with the correct formula and constants developed for that population (Lohman, 1984). For example, in samples of adult males and females over 50 years of age, no formulas for converting body density (D_b) to percent fat have been developed to replace the Siri formula:

$$\% \text{ Fat} = \left(\frac{4.95}{D_b} - 4.50 \right) 100.$$

Because the water content of the fat-free body may be decreasing, increasing, or not changing, between the ages of 50 and 90, it is at present uncertain how to adjust the Siri formula for the decreasing proportion of mineral in the fat-free body with an unknown water change. This problem is addressed briefly at the end of chapter 6 and is presently being addressed by several ongoing research investigations on other populations as well.

The Need for New Reference Methods

New reference methods are greatly needed to obtain more direct estimates of muscle, bone, and fat as well as to estimate regional body composition. The development of dual energy radiography (chapter 3) and total body electrical conductivity measurement (chapter 11) may complement densitometry and hydrometry as the four major laboratory methods for validation studies. However, whether any of these methods will be shown to have prediction errors less than 2% fat within a given population remains to be determined. I predict that the density-water combined approaches (and other multicomponent models) will become widely accepted, along with total body electrical conductivity and dual energy radiography, as the leading body composition methodologies in the 1990s. In addition, the development of regional body composition assessment will be a prominent area of investigation in the field in the coming years.

Regional Estimates of Body Composition

Although the field of body composition has emphasized total body composition and its relation to health, a shift is taking place as new methodologies are developed to estimate regional composition allowing analysis of the independent contributions of regional and total body composition to health. In the 1990s we must emphasize the study of regional assessment and its biological significance. Dual energy radiography and segmental impedance offer promise in this area, as do anthropometry, computed tomography, and magnetic resonance imaging.

Population-Specific Body Composition Equations

Once body composition can be more accurately assessed in various populations with new reference methods or with more accurate multicomponent approaches, then better population-specific anthropometric equations can be developed for use in schools (chapter 9), pediatrics, weight loss clinics, and hospital, fitness, and sports medicine settings (chapter 10) on such populations as the acute and chronically ill, male and female athletes, children (chapter 6), the elderly, and populations at high risk for chronic diseases. Anthropometry will remain useful in these settings for assessing total and regional body composition, complementing the development of new methodologies.

Summary

In this chapter I have presented a brief perspective on the developing field of body composition assessment, a short overview of basic concepts, a review of the problems of terminology, the frame of reference for a validation scale, the need for new reference methods in addition to densitometry, the development of regional body composition assessment, and the use of new anthropometric equations tied to these new developments. The lack of a common approach to these concepts has hindered the development of the field and contributed to redundancy of efforts. A greater diversity of research goals emphasizing a common framework is needed.

Chapter 2

Body Density, Body Water, and Bone Mineral: Controversies and Limitations of the Two-Component System

Densitometry and hydrometry are two of the criterion methods often used in validation studies of new body composition methods. Estimating body composition from either method is based on the assumption that body water and mineral content as a fraction of fat-free body are essentially constant from day to day, for a given individual as well as among individuals. But controversy exists among investigators about the extent to which this is true. Dissatisfaction with the two-component system has led to the development of multicomponent models in the search for more accurate assessment of body composition in terms of adipose, muscle, and bone (or fat, water, and mineral).

S ome experts still view body density as the gold standard for measurement of body composition, whereas others are critical of its use in validation studies of new methods because variation in body density independent of fatness is associated with variation in water, protein, and mineral content. A third group, including me, believe that densitometry remains a useful standard within many populations, especially young adult males and females, but that population-specific equations need to replace the general use of the Siri (1961) and Brozek et al. (1963) equations.

$$\text{Siri: \% Fat} = \left(\frac{4.95}{D_b} - 4.50 \right) 100$$

$$\text{Brozek: \% Fat} = \left(\frac{4.570}{D_b} - 4.142 \right) 100$$

Furthermore, we favor the use of body water content along with body density rather than density alone to estimate body fatness, as Siri (1956) first proposed:

7

$$\% \text{ Fat} = \left(\frac{2.118}{D_b} - 0.78 \, w - 1.354 \right) 100,$$

where w = the fraction of water in the body.

Alternatively, when the mineral content of the body (m) can be estimated, we would use the formula of Lohman (1986), which is derived later in this chapter:

$$\% \text{ Fat} = \left(\frac{6.386}{D_b} + 3.961 \, m - 6.090 \right) 100.$$

These and other multicomponent approaches are in need of further development if body density measurements are to more accurately estimate body fatness. It was Siri (1956) who, because of variation in water and in the protein-to-mineral ratio of the fat-free body mass, proposed a 4% error (standard deviation) in body fatness estimates from densitometry in the general population (a mixture of all ages, activity levels, and ethnic groups). In 1961, Siri estimated that a variability of 2% for body water will lead to a 2.7% fat error (0.0057 g/cc) and that a variability in the protein-to-mineral ratio will lead to a 2.1% fat error (0.0046 g/cc). He also estimated two additional sources of error related to variation in the composition of adipose tissue, which together lead to a 1.9% fat error (0.0040 g/cc) in the general population. By adding the squares of the standard deviations, (2.7, 2.1, and 1.9) and taking the square root of the sum, we can estimate the total error from the three sources combined (using the law of propagation of errors to be 3.9%).

Estimating Fat-Free Body Composition

Bakker and Struikenkamp (1977) examined the source of variation in the density of lean body mass from an anatomical as well as a chemical basis. From a review of the related literature, they found results similar to those of Siri (1961) for the effects of water variability of LBM, with an estimated 2% body water in the general population, causing a variation in the LBM density of 0.008 g/cc. Then they examined the skeleton and its contribution to variation in the LBM density, first by assuming a constant density and looking only at the effect of variation in the skeletal fraction of the LBM and then looking at estimates of the variation of the density of the skeleton. Together, these two sources of variation would cause a variability of 0.003 g/cc in the LBM density. Finally, according to Bakker and Struikenkamp (1977), they examined the variation in the fat-free adipose tissue content of LBM and estimated a 0.002 g/cc variability from the source. Adding all four sources gives a result similar to that of Siri (1961). If these estimates are correct for a representative sample of subjects of all ages and various ethnic groups and activity levels, we can see that densitometry is not an ideal method for such validation studies as that by Segal, Gutin, Presta, Wang, and Van Itallie (1985), where a wide age range of subjects was used and where the standard errors of estimate from various methods are 5% or greater, using densitometry as the criterion. I contend that density needs to be adjusted for variation in water and mineral contents before it can be used as a criterion in subjects over 55 years of age. This recommendation is contrary to the practice of many research validation studies.

A recent example of the misuse of the two-component model over a wide age range is the work of Pierson et al. (1991). These investigators compared densitometry with all the major methods of estimating body composition in a sample of subjects ranging from young adults to the elderly and reported a translation table allowing one to convert an estimate of fatness by one method to another. Unfortunately, the conversion equations are highly dependent on age of subject, because of changes in fat-free body composition with age, and this was entirely ignored in the equation published.

What about variation in water and mineral contents of fat-free body in a more specific population homogeneous for age, gender, and ethnicity? In previous work I estimated that one half of the variance of the fat-free body density in the general population would be found within a specific population and that the combined effect of the major sources of variation would lead to an error of 2.77% (Table 2.1) and a variation in the density of the fat-free body of 0.0059 g/cc (Lohman, 1981).

Therefore, percent-fat error within a specific population, because of biological variation in the density of the fat-free body for the three major sources, is

$$\% \text{ Fat error} = \sqrt{.(1.9)^2 + (1.5)^2 + (1.35)^2} = 2.77\%.$$

Two observations reinforce these estimates. One is by Womersley and Durnin (1977) where they suggest that one half of the variation between skinfolds and densitometry should be assigned to each method. A second observation is that when skinfolds are used to predict body density (based on 12 studies; Lohman, 1981) in the young adult male, the average standard error of estimation (SEE) is 0.0070 g/cc. Dividing this error in half gives a variation of 0.0049 g/cc to body density and 0.0049 g/cc to skinfolds.

Thus, this indirect empirical way of attributing variation between two methods to variation in the fat-free body density is in close agreement with the more

Table 2.1   Hypothesized Variation in Body Density With Variation in Fat-Free Body Composition in a Specific Population

Source of variation	Density, g/cc	% Fat error
Water	0.0040	1.90
Protein/mineral	0.0033	1.50
Obesity composition	0.0029	1.35

theoretical estimates provided by Siri (1961), Bakker and Struikenkamp (1977), and Lohman (1981). This analysis has been overlooked by those who criticize body density as a criterion variable and argue that densitometry is not a valid measure of composition from which to evaluate new methods. The use of densitometry is not a perfect method, but its use in the young adult population serves adequately as a method to evaluate other methods, provided the researchers keep in mind an inherent error of ± 2.0% to 2.8% fat in that population. This error is probably larger for children and the elderly, where variation in water and mineral contents with growth and aging add variability to the 0.0059 g/cc young adult estimate, as is suggested by the cadaver analysis of older people done by Clarys, Martin, and Drinkwater (1984) and Martin, Drinkwater, Clarys, and Ross (1986). Unfortunately only anatomical and no chemical data have been published in this research. The authors' effort to generalize the variability found in the elderly to young adults overlooks the large body of empirical evidence showing the usefulness of densitometry in developing skinfold and bioelectric impedance equations in the young and middle-aged adult.

Precision Versus Accuracy: Densitometry

The previous section dealt with the variation in body density due to three biological sources: fat, water, and mineral. Due to variation in the water and mineral contents of the fat-free body, the interpretation of body density as an index of body fatness leads to errors of 2% to 4%, depending on the population being studied. Now I will focus on the measurement of body density from underwater weighing, which also contributes to the error in estimating body fatness. How precisely (repeatable) and how accurately (how close to the actual value) can body density be measured? If the portion of biological variation in body density associated with variation in the density of fat-free body mass is 0.0059 g/cc as estimated in the previous section, what is the additional variation associated with technical error?

Akers and Buskirk (1969) analyzed the major sources of variation in body density measurement. Variation in residual lung volume was the largest source of variation. Variation in body weight, underwater weighing, and the measurement of water temperature at the time of underwater weight are much smaller, having a combined error of 0.0006 g/cc if body weight is measured within 0.02 kg, underwater weight within 0.02 kg, and water temperature within 0.0005 degrees. The combined error from residual volume, when estimated within 100 ml (equivalent to a 0.00139-g/cc variation in body density) by oxygen dilution procedure (Wilmore, 1969) and the above sources, is 0.0015 g/ml, or 0.7% fat. Variation in body density of 0.0015 to 0.0020 g/ml is characteristic of trial-to-trial variation within a given day, reflecting the combined measurement error inherent in most underwater weighing systems. Within-subject standard deviations larger than 0.0020 g/ml reflect larger measurement errors in one or more of the components of body density and indicate a need to improve the measurement precision. It is essential that each laboratory using an underwater weighing system conduct periodic estimates of intrasubject variation, using 10 or more subjects, each measured three or more times. Additional sources of variation in body density determinations are apparent when between-day within-subject estimations of technical error are carried out. The results of such studies indicate a technical error of 0.003 g/cc (Jackson, Pollock, Graves, & Mahar, 1988), equivalent to 1.1% fat in men and 1.2% fat in women.

The sources of this additional error are likely to be associated with day-to-day variation in the water content of the body rather than technical measurement error and variation in the volume of gas in the gastrointestinal tract, which is usually assumed to be a constant volume of 100 ml for all subjects. Little day-to-day variation is expected in fat, protein, or mineral content of the body over a 7- to 10-day period. In summary, we can see that the technical error of estimation of body density is quite small when residual volume is measured (this is not the case where residual volume is estimated from height and weight, where errors between 300 and 400 ml can easily occur for a given subject; Lohman, 1981) and when other sources of variation are precisely measured. Thus, the precision of this method is such that percent fat can be determined with a technical error of less than 1%. The accuracy of the measurement of body density, however, is another matter. It depends on carefully calibrated systems for body weight, underwater weight, and residual volume determination. Interlaboratory comparisons of the same subjects have been used to help identify systematic differences among laboratories associated with calibration errors. If variation across laboratories is greater than 0.0015 g/cc for the same subject, we must be suspicious. As part of an interlaboratory study to evaluate the validity of the bioelectric impedance method (chapter 4), the results shown in Table 2.2 were found for seven laboratories, each measuring the same two subjects for body density. For each subject a standard deviation of 0.0015 g/cc was found, indicating that the between-laboratory variation was within the acceptable range.

Hydrometry as a Method of Estimating Body Fatness

In their review article on the measurement of total body water, Schoeller, Kushner, Dietz, and Bandini (1985) outline the major approaches and methodologies for determination of body water content using isotope dilution techniques. Siri (1961) presents arguments for the use of the water content of the human body as a method of estimating body fatness (f, or fraction of body weight as fat) from total body water estimates and the proportion of water in the fat-free body:

$$f = 1 - w/w'$$

where w is the measured total body water in liters and w' is the proportion of water in the fat-free body. Sources of variation in w' are (a) variation in the hydration level of a given subject from day to day, (b) variation in the proportion of water in the fat-free body from population to population (e.g., children vs. adults, males vs. female, obese vs. lean, and elderly vs. young adult), and (c) variation in the water content of adipose tissue associated with greater levels of

Table 2.2 Interlaboratory Comparisons for Densitometry, Body Weight, and Whole-Body Resistance for BIA

Subject 1	Laboratory							
	A	C	D	E	G	H	X	S
Body density, g/cc	1.0609	1.0609	1.0589	1.0631	1.0600	—	1.0608	0.0015
Body weight, kg	52.4	52.5	52.3	51.8	52.8	—	52.4	0.36
Body resistance, ohms	510	532	528	521	516	—	529	8.9

Subject 2	Laboratory							
	A	C	D	E	G	H	X	S
Body density, g/cc	1.067	1.0688	1.0677	1.0679	1.0660	1.0650	1.0670	0.0014
Body weight, kg	78.1	78.3	78.3	78.3	78.1	79.6	78.6	0.57
Body resistance, ohms	385	400	382	376	389	399	389	9.5

body fatness. Siri (1961) estimates that if there were no technical error in the measurement of body water, there still would remain an error in the estimation of percent fat of 3.6% associated with biological variability in the water content of the fat-free body (2%). It can be argued that, in a specific population measured in the fasted state, the water content variation may be less than 2% extended by Siri (1961), thus theoretical errors are given in Table 2.3 for 1%, 1.5%, and 2.0% variation in water content of the body. For example, if reference body (Brozek et al., 1963) is increased from 62.4% water content to 63.9%, the percent fat would decrease from 15.3% to 13.4%, or a 1.9% error.

The calculations in Table 2.3 are based on the formula $F = 1 - w/w'$ and not on the error analysis as developed by Siri (1961) for the general population. Thus, in a specific population, such as adult women, a 2% variation in body water content (percentage of body weight) corresponds to a percent-fat error of 2.6% based on the above formula as compared to a 3.6% fat error in the general population based on Siri's error analysis. Important to the controversy of using body water as a criterion method for estimating body composition is the empirical evidence that supports or refutes its use. In a study to validate bioelectric impedance (Van Loan et al., 1990), both body water content and body density were measured in 150 young adults, and a correlation of .97 was found between FFB estimated from densitometry (FFB_d) and FFB estimated from body water (FFB_w). The standard error of estimate for the prediction of (FFB_d) from (FFB_w) was 2.7 kg, as compared to 2.5 kg from (FFB_d) predicted from bioelectric impedance and 3.7 kg predicting (FFB_w) from bioelectrical impedance (Van Loan, Boileau, Christ, et al., 1990). In this study the 2.7-kg error in predicting (FFB_d) from body water yields a SEE for percent fat of 4.5% between methods—much larger than expected from Table 2.3. Part of this variation is interlaboratory variation in total body water determinations, and part may be within-laboratory technical error in measuring body water, rather than biological variation. The work of Young, Bogan, Roe, and Lutevak (1968) also implies large biological or technical variation in measuring body water in their work,

Table 2.3 Variation in Body Water Content and Corresponding Percent-Fat Errors From Body Water Determination in a Specific Population

Changes in body water content	Water content (W)	W/FFB	% Fat error
Reference body (RB)	62.4	73.8	0
RB + 1.0%	63.4	74.9	1.2
RB + 1.5%	63.9	75.5	1.9
RB + 2.0%	64.4	76.0	2.5

Reference body weight is 65.3 kg with a 62.4% water content and a 73.8% fat-free body water content (Brozek et al., 1963).

with low association found between water content and body composition in an adolescent sample. Upon reanalysis of the data, I found (Lohman, 1986) a decrease in their subject's water content as a fraction of fat-free body mass with age when a multicomponent model (water and density) was used to estimate fat-free body mass.

Precision Versus Accuracy: Hydrometry

The use of total body water to estimate body fat and fat-free body content until recently has been overlooked by many laboratories as a criterion method, primarily because of methodological problems. Body water is estimated from isotope dilution procedures using deuterium oxide (^2H_2O—heavy water), tritium oxide (^3H_2O—radioactive water), or $H_2^{18}O$ as tracers. The nonradioactive isotope deuterium can be measured by infrared absorptiometry or mass spectroscopy. The critical methodological concerns with the isotope dilution technique relate to (a) the accuracy and precision of estimates obtained when different physiological fluids are sampled and (b) the magnitude of the protein-hydrogen exchangeability. The critical biological concerns relate to (a) the constancy of hydration of fat-free body and source of variation within a given population, such as menstrual cycle, dehydration from exercise, and dehydration from drugs or disease, and (b) the mean hydration of the fat-free body as a function of population, including, for example, the elderly, prepubescent children, and infants.

The sources of technical error for estimating body water from the isotope dilution approach include choice of physiological fluid (saliva, urine, blood, respiratory water), equilibration time of the isotopic tracers, loss of isotope during the equilibration period, correction for the isotopic dilution space (deuterium dilution space in larger than 18_O dilution space), correction for the protein-hydrogen exchangeable fraction, and choice of analytical method for determining the isotope concentration after equilibration has been reached. Each of these sources is discussed by Schoeller et al. (1985), and more recently these authors have made a case for standardization of body water measurements (Schoeller & Jones, 1987) by proposing standard procedures and calculations for all body water measurements. Because these sources of error are present to different degrees according to the choices made by each investigator, each study has a characteristic technical error, which often has not been estimated. Respiratory water sampling is the most practical choice of physiological fluid, because of sample purity and noninvasive sampling, so it is essential that future investigators determine the precision and accuracy of this approach. Schoeller et al. (1985) have indicated that, because isotopically labeled water has a lower vapor pressure than unlabeled water, this approach may lead to an overestimation of total body water unless the fractionalization effect is estimated. Also, atmospheric moisture can be drawn into the trapped breath water during the 10-minute collection period, causing a change in the isotope fractionalization. Secondly, the use of infrared spectrometry is less expensive than mass spectrometry for measuring isotope enrichment; however, mass spectrometry is the most precise method.

Based on the work of Schoeller et al. (1985), in a comparison of five individuals measured twice over a 14-day period, the body water ratio varied by 2%. This intrasubject variation needs to be established by each laboratory, using body water techniques as a criterion variable. In the seven males investigated by Bunt, Lohman, and Boileau (1989), a 1.1% standard deviation was estimated in the water content of fat-free body within subjects measured two times, 3 weeks apart. It may be that much of the variation in interinvestigator results using total body water comes about because of technical errors that increase the standard deviation to 2 to 3 times the expected value of 1% to 2%.

Body Density and Water Content

Because of limitations in the two-component approach for accurate estimation of body composition, various multicomponent approaches have been developed where two or more constituents of the body are measured. Such approaches enable, theoretically, a more accurate estimate of body composition than the two-component approach, where only one component, such as body density, is measured. For example, Siri (1956, 1961) put forth one of the first multicomponent approaches when he derived the theoretical relation between percent fat, body density, and body water shown in the following equation:

$$\% \text{ Fat} = \left(\frac{2.118}{D_b} - 0.78\ w - 1.354 \right) 100.$$

He assumed that the ratio of mineral to protein (5 to 12) in the fat-free body and density of the solids (1.565 g/cc) are constant. The above equation was derived from the more general equation:

$$\frac{1}{D_b} = \frac{f}{d_f} + \frac{w}{d_w} + \frac{p}{d_p} + \frac{m}{d_m}$$

where d_f, d_w, d_p, and d_m equal the respective densities of fat, water, protein, and mineral, and, f, w, p, and m equal the fraction of body weight as fat, water, protein, and mineral.

As long as the fat-free solids remain constant in composition and density, this multicomponent model applies to several populations and should serve populations of both children and adults. According to Siri's estimates, the use of this equation would decrease the percent-fat error from 4% based on body density alone to 2% for density and water. This proposed major reduction in error has yet to be taken advantage of in most body composition validation studies. Recently, however, Van Loan, Boileau, Christ, et al. (1990), Houtkooper, Lohman, et al. (1989), and Slaughter et al. (1988) compared density versus water versus water-density equations as three criterion methods to validate anthropometric and bioelectric impedance. In all cases the prediction errors are reduced by the use of such multicomponent criterion methods over the two-component model.

Using the Siri water-density equation, we can show advantages in the same subject at two states of hydration over density alone. Using body density alone, Bunt et al. (1989) found that the mean body density in seven women measured at a time in their menstrual cycle when their body weight was at its lowest (body weight = 58.9 kg) was 1.0430 g/cc, as compared to a body density of 1.0370 g/cc when their body weight was highest during their cycle (weight = 61.1 kg). Percent fat changed from 24.8% to 27.6%, based on the two-component model (Table 2.4). For this study, only females with regular menstrual cycles who experienced considerable weight fluctuation were recruited. For 4 weeks prior to the study, day-to-day fluctuations in body weight were monitored, and the timing of low and high points in body weight were observed. This research design differed from that of Byrd and Thomas (1983), who found no significant change in body density in 12 females measured at preselected times for two consecutive cycles. The small changes in body weight found in their sample suggest that body water changes in many females are too small to detect by present methodology. In the Bunt et al. (1989) study, the 2.2-kg change in body weight was over 6 times larger than the average change observed in the Byrd and Thomas study. Percent fat, using the Siri water-density formula, increased from 22.7% to 24.2% and was larger than expected based on theoretical calculation of the change in body density associated with a change in total body water of 2.2 kg, assuming all the change in body weight was due to an increase in body water. The expected value of body density for the subjects at the heavier weight was 1.0408 g/cc, whereas the actual value was 1.0370 g/cc. This discrepancy has yet to be explained, and this study needs to be repeated in another group of subjects with additional measures of composition to determine possible reasons for the discrepancy. The results are shown in Figure 2.1 for each subject, where the changes in body density ranged from 0.001 to 0.010 g/cc as compared to that predicted by the

Table 2.4   Changes in Estimated Fat Content Based on Variation in Body Density During the Menstrual Cycle in Seven Women

Item	Body weight	Body density	Body water, L	Body fat, kg	% Water	% Fat
Low weight, kg	58.9	1.0434	33.6	14.5	57.7	24.7
Expect values with 2.2 kg increase	61.1	1.0408	35.8	14.5	59.3	25.6
High weight, kg	61.1	1.0370	35.1	16.9	57.7	27.6

Note. Data from Bunt et al. (1989, p. 98).

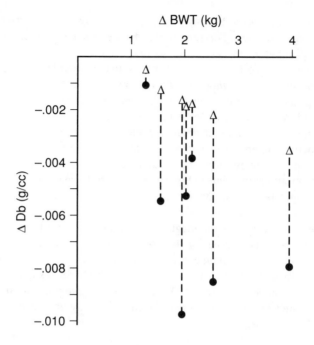

Figure 2.1   Relationship of individual increases in body weight (ΔBWT) versus decreases in body density (ΔDb) of female subjects (*N* = 7). *Note.* From J.C. Bunt, T.G. Lohman, and R.A. Boileau, "Impact of Total Body Water Fluctuation on Estimating of Body Fat from Body Density," *Medicine and Science in Sports and Exercise,* **21,** pp. 96-100, 1989, © by the American College of Sports Medicine. Adapted by permission.

changes in body water, assuming all differences in weight were due to body water (Bunt et al., 1989).

Body Density and Mineral Content

The mineral content of the fat-free mass in reference body (Brozek et al., 1963) was estimated to be 6.8% on the basis of four male cadavers. With the development of dual energy X-ray absorptiometry (chapter 3), total bone mineral can be estimated in living children, adults, and the aged. The biological variation in the mineral content in various populations can now be estimated, and reference values can be developed using dual energy X-ray absorptiometry (DEXA)-derived bone estimates. The relationship between bone mineral and total body mineral is important to document, so that accurate estimates of total mineral content can be made from bone mineral estimates provided by DEXA. Brozek et al. (1963) estimated that osseous mineral represents 82.4% of total body mineral, based on careful analysis of limited data on cadavers in the literature. Heymsfield, Wang, Kehayias, Heshka, et al. (1989) estimate both the osseous and the nonosseous mineral content using a four-compartment model, using neutron activation analysis, hydrometry, and DPA methodologies, and indicate that 87% of total body mineral is osseous bone mineral. They found the total mineral content of five males ranging from 42 to 94 years of age to be 6.1% of FFB; for eight females ranging from 24 to 85 years of age, the mean mineral content was 6.4%. Other estimates of the mineral content of the body reviewed in chapter 3 indicate that the magnitude in male-female differences in mineral content and reference value for the young adult population is uncertain at the present time. The development of an appropriate reference value for each population would allow us more accurate body-fat estimation from the densitometry method. Figure 2.2 illustrates the possible populations that need to be investigated to establish reference values for body composition assessment.

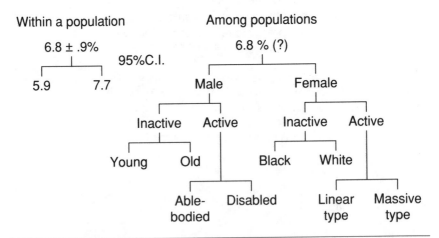

Figure 2.2   Biological variation in the mineral content of fat-free body among populations. *Note.* Reprinted with permision of Ross Laboratories, Columbus, OH 43216, from *Body Composition Assessment in Youth and Adults,* © 1985 by Ross Laboratories.

The effect of varying the mineral content of the body on estimated percent fat can be determined using the density-mineral formula I developed (Lohman, 1986). Taking the Siri water-density formula derivation (1956),

$$\% \text{ Fat} = \frac{d_f}{d_s - d_f} \left[\frac{d_f}{D_b} - w \left(\frac{d_s - d_w}{d_w} \right) - 1.0 \right] 100,$$

where

d_s = the density of solid (protein and mineral)
d_w = the density of water
d_f = density of fat
w = water as a fraction of body weight.

One can obtain the water-density results of

$$\% \text{ Fat} = \left(\frac{2.118}{D_b} - 0.78 \, w - 1.354 \right) 100.$$

A similar approach can be used to derive an equation for estimating body fat from body density and mineral. If

$$\% \text{ Fat} = \frac{d_f}{d_{pw} - d_f} \left[\frac{d_{pw}}{D_b} - m \left(\frac{d_{pw} - d_m}{d_m} \right) - 1.0 \right] 100,$$

then

$$\% \text{ Fat} = \left(\frac{6.386}{D_b} + 3.961 \, m - 6.090 \right) 100,$$

where

d_b = density of the whole body
d_f = density of fat = 0.9007 g/cc
d_s = density of mineral = 3.037 g/cc
d_w = density of water = 0.99007 g/cc
d_{pw} = density of protein + water = 1.0486
w = water as a fraction of body weight
m = mineral as a fraction of body weight.

Table 2.5 shows how, using this formula in the female population, percent-fat estimates would change by varying the mineral content of the body at a given body density.

A second way to account for the effect of bone mineral on body fat estimates is with the use of multiple regression and the development of empirical formulas as illustrated by my work with children (Lohman, Slaugher, Boileau, Bunt, &

Table 2.5   Theoretical Estimates of Percent Fat Varying the Body Mineral Content Using the Density-Mineral Formula and a Constant Body Density = 1.040 g/cc

Mineral content body (%)	% Fat[a]
4.0	20.9
4.5	22.9
5.0	24.8
5.5	26.8
6.0	28.8

[a]Percent fat calculated from $\left(\dfrac{6.386}{D_b} + 3.961\ m - 6.090 \right) 100.$

Lussier, 1984) and forearm bone mineral, and Bunt et al. (1990) and Going, Pamenter, Lohman, Carswell, Westfall, Perry, and Boyden (1990) with spine and forearm bone mineral. In the latter case, in a sample of athletic females, we found the following equation to be associated with body density:

$$D_b = 0.00063\ \Sigma SK + 0.0155\ L2\text{-}4_{BMC} + 0.0252\ RS_{BMC} + 1.0460.$$

From this equation we estimated the effect of varying radius and spine bone mineral on percent-fat estimates in various athletic groups (Bunt et al., 1990). In the research of Going et al. (1990), we adjusted body density for varying levels of spine and radius bone mineral content for each individual before correlating estimates of body fat from dual photon absorptiometry and densitometry. The use of total body bone mineral to adjust percent-fat estimates should yield even better estimates of body fat than the use of regional bone mineral estimates and allow us to determine the actual magnitude of densitometric error of percent-fat estimates in various populations with above- or below-average bone mineral content. Thus, if the total mineral content of an individual is known or can be assumed to be close to the population mean for him or her, then a correction can be applied to the density–percent-fat formulas to prevent underestimation of fatness for individuals with above-average amounts of bone mineral and overestimation of fatness from body density for those with below-average amounts of bone.

We can see how this variation in bone mineral can be a significant problem in determining minimal weight in a very lean athlete whose percent fat is being estimated from body density. With a density of 1.0903 g/cc and a mineral content of the fat-free body (6.5% of body weight) of 6.8%, one's fat content will be estimated at 4.0% using either the Siri formula

$$\% \text{ Fat} = \left(\frac{4.95}{D_b} - 4.50 \right) 100$$

or the Lohman (1986) mineral-density formula

$$\% \text{ Fat} = \left(\frac{6.386}{D_b} + 3.961 \, m - 6.090 \right) 100.$$

However, if the mineral content is increased to 7.4% of body weight (7.7% of the fat-free body) and body fatness is held constant, then body density would increase to 1.094 g/cc. If the mineral content is decreased to 5.7% of the body (5.9% of fat-free body) while holding body fatness constant, then body density would be 1.0813 g/cc. The estimate of mineral of 6.8% ± 0.9% is the 95% confidence interval I proposed within a given population (Lohman, 1985, see Figure 2.2). This variation is of some controversy, with a much greater variation being proposed on the basis of cadaver work in an elderly sample (Martin et al., 1986) using an anatomic model.

Biological Sources of Bone Mineral: Genetics and the Environment

Important to the area of bone mineral estimation is the quantification of genetic, activity, dietary, and hormonal influences in both the developing and the aging populations. There are two major sources of variation in the mineral content of the fat-free body. One is that some individuals inherit or develop a larger frame size relative to their height than others. These individuals will tend to have a higher FFB mineral content than those with a smaller frame size. A second source of variation is that some individuals inherit or develop a denser skeleton than average and thus also have a higher mineral content. These two sources of variation may be related or independent of each other, and until we can actually measure bone density (g/cc) with low radiation exposure, estimates of the contribution of each factor will be difficult to assess.

Because of the importance of bone development in the prevention of osteoporosis, it will be important to better identify the relative role of genetics versus environment factors influencing both skeletal size and bone mineral density (g/cc). The review article by Pollitzer and Anderson (1989) shows the important influences of genetic and ethnic factors, along with dietary and activity factors, in explaining bone mass differences in the population at large. It may be that the genetic component will be greater than any of the other environmental contributors, as genetics affects skeletal size and bone density more than do dietary history, activity history, gender and ethnic background, or other contributors of mineral content in the fat-free body. However, we are a long way yet from sorting out these factors and their relative contributions.

The Multicomponent Model: Density, Water Content, and Mineral Content

A theoretical model can be developed to predict body fatness from the combination of body density, body water content, and mineral content of the body. A student of mine, Dr. Arie Selinger, first derived this formula in his dissertation research at the University of Illinois in 1977 (Selinger, 1977), extending Siri's work with water and density:

$$\% \text{ Fat} = \left(\frac{2.747}{D_b} - 0.714\ w + 1.129b + 1.222\ m - 1.027 \right) 100.$$

Substituting into the formula the densities of water (w, 0.9937 g/cc), protein (p, 1.34 g/cc), osseous mineral (b, 2.982 g/cc), nonosseous mineral (m, 3.317 g/cc), and fat (f, 0.9007 g/cc), the equation becomes

$$\% \text{ Fat} = \left(\frac{2.747}{D_b} - 0.714\ w + 1.146b - 2.0503 \right) 100,$$

assuming the m (nonosseous mineral) increase is proportional to b (osseous mineral).

The equation applies to any age group and thus is not population specific, provided that the densities of protein and mineral are reasonably constant for all age and ethnic groups. From a theoretical standpoint, body fatness can be estimated more accurately using this multicomponent approach than by using a two-component approach, provided that the density, water content, and mineral content of the body can be accurately and precisely measured. With the use of DEXA as a measure of total bone mineral (b), this equation is likely to be used a great deal more in the future and may become a better criterion method for future validation studies. In our work with skinfolds and percent fat estimated from this multicomponent approach, we found closer association with percent fat from this model than with percent fat from density alone in a large sample of growing children (Slaughter et al., 1988).

Summary

In this chapter we have investigated the multicomponent model of body density, body water content, and mineral content in an attempt to overcome some of the limitations of the two-component model, which assumes a constant density and composition of the fat-free body mass. The variation in water and mineral contents of the fat-free body was explored to better highlight the controversy around the assumed constancy of fat-free body composition. Technical errors were defined for various methods to show the highly precise methodologies needed to solve the multicomponent questions. With the impact of variation in water and mineral content on body density well described from a theoretical perspective, emphasis is given to the shortcomings of empirical data to support theoretical calculations.

Although body density is no longer the standard for body composition assessment, it remains a valuable tool, when properly used, for assessment of body composition and evaluation of new methodologies. Further research utilizing the density-water, density-mineral, and density-water-mineral approaches offers promise of more accurate assessment of body composition in validation studies as well as a check on quality control of data methodological precision. The improvement of these multicomponent approaches, along with promising new methodologies such as dual energy radiography (chapter 3) and total body electrical conductivity (chapter 11) to assess body composition, will characterize research effects in the early 1990s to develop better criterion approaches to the study of body composition.

Dual Energy Radiography: Total Body and Regional Composition

With the development of dual energy radiography, total body and regional composition, including bone mineral content and the fat and lean contents of the soft tissue, can be estimated with a very low radiation exposure and more precise measurement than was previously possible. The question at issue is whether more accurate body composition assessment in growth and development and aging studies can be attained and whether this new method will gain recognition as a reference method for future body composition validation studies.

The development of dual photon absorptiometry (DPA) using [153]Gd (Ross & Skoldborn, 1974) enabled measurement of spine and femur bone mineral content (g/cm and g/cm^2), as compared to single photon absorptiometry (SPA), which was limited to bone mineral assessment on the radius and ulna. This dual energy technique was later extended to total body absorptiometry and the estimation of total bone mineral content (Mazess, Peppler, & Gibbons, 1984; Mazess, Peppler, Chestnut, Nelp, & Cohn, 1981). Except for neutron activation analysis, the DPA approach is the first to provide researchers with the long-awaited technology to study variation in bone mineral content of the body. In addition to obtaining estimates of bone mineral, Mazess et al. (1984) found that the dual energy approach could also be used to estimate the fat and lean contents of the soft tissue of the body. Thus, this new technique to furnish total body composition was put forth. Further testing of DPA in comparison with other body composition methods yielded standard errors of prediction for fat content between 3.2% and 4.7% (Heymsfield, Wang, Kehayias, & Pierson, 1989).

In 1987 the first commercially available dual energy X-ray absorptiometer (DEXA) was designed to estimate spine bone mineral content with greater precision and less radiation exposure than DPA. By 1989, three different commercially available absorptiometers using X-ray rather than gamma-ray radiation were developed with the capability of measuring total body, as well as regional, composition. Comparisons between DPA and the new X-ray technologies have shown good agreement, with the lower scanning times and increased precision characteristic of the new technique (Gluer et al., 1990).

Bone Mineral Assessment

Because of the rapid development of this field, the terminology has not yet been standardized, and several names represent the same technique, though the instruments may differ in technical aspects (Gluer et al., 1990). For this chapter, a *bone densitometer* is any instrument that uses gamma rays or X-rays to estimate bone mineral content (g/cm) and bone mineral density (g/cm^2). Because bone area, but not volume, can be estimated by these instruments, bone density (g/cm^3) cannot be measured; however, by convention in this field, bone mineral density (BMD, sometimes called areal density) has been defined as g/cm^2.

Early in the development of this field, bone densitometry was limited to single photon absorptiometers (SPA) with 125-Iodine serving as a source of gamma radiation. This approach enabled precise measurement of the bone mineral content (BMC) and bone mineral density (BMD) of the radius and ulna, but not of other parts of the body. Using this technique in children and young adults, our work and that of others found changes in the bone mineral content of the fat-free body with maturation in children and youth (see chapter 6).

The dual photon absorptiometer (^{153}Gd) enabled estimates of spine and femur and, in time, total body bone mineral. With the development of dual energy X-ray sources of radiation, new technologies were developed, and several acronyms appeared, including *DEXA* (dual energy X-ray absorptiometry), *DRA* (dual energy radiographic absorptiometry), *DER* (dual energy radiography), and *QDR* (quantitative digital radiography). The relationship among these technologies is shown in Figure 3.1.

DPA Versus DER: Short- and Long-Term Precision

Limitations in the precision of DPA, particularly in the areas of assessing changes in bone mineral over time and estimating the fat content of the soft tissue, have

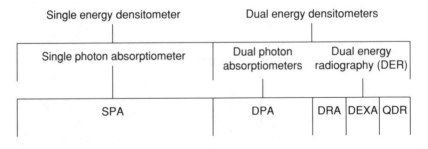

Figure 3.1   Bone densitometers.

opened the way for the replacement of this relatively new technology by dual energy radiography (DER). Not only has DPA shown greater variability than is optimal (Mazess, Barden, Bisek, & Hansen, 1990; Gluer et al., 1990), but the problems of source decay and replacement for DPA add to a further loss of precision over the long term (Gluer et al., 1990). With DER, one X-ray source yields a relatively constant radiation dose over the long term, eliminating the problem of this source of decay associated with DPA.

The short-term precision of DER has recently been described by Mazess et al. (1990) for whole-body and regional estimates of lean, bone, mineral, and fat, based on 10 repeated measurements on each of 12 subjects (2 measurements per day) over a 5- to 7-day period. The authors reported the coefficients of variation (CVs) for BMC and BMD of the total body to be 1.5% and 0.6%. For the lean in the soft tissue (g), the CV was 1.6%. For percent fat in the soft tissue, the precision of measurement (standard deviation) was 1.2%, similar to the results of Jackson, Pollock, Graves, and Mahar (1988) for the reliability of percent fat from underwater weighing, skinfold, and bioelectric impedance (see chapter 4). When bone mineral mass (g) was expressed as a percent of fat-free soft tissue mass, a mean of 5.8% was found with a precision of 0.13% (CV = 2.3%). This small amount of variation is remarkable and offers a precision of obtaining bone mineral content of the fat-free body never before available.

Long-term precision of DER and DPA has been investigated using phantoms. Results by Gluer et al. (1990) on the spine phantom show less variation for DER than for DPA (0.44 vs. 1.4 CV). The CVs for the whole-body BMD on one skeleton was 0.4% for 34 determinations on 1 DER scanner and less than 1% among 37 scanners (Mazess et al., 1990). In our work using DER in 104 adult women, we found the total bone mineral (g/cm^2) to have a CV of 1.4% on retesting all subjects 7 to 10 days after the initial test (Hansen et al., in press).

Whole-Body Composition From DER

The use of bone densitometries for determination of whole-body composition was first developed on DPA and then extended to DER. Theoretical bases for obtaining both bone estimates of the whole body and fat content of soft tissue were first described by Peppler and Mazess (1981). Because R_{ST} (the attenuation coefficient over soft tissue reflects the relative lean and soft content) differs greatly from R_B (the attenuation coefficient while the bone is being scanned), the attenuation coefficient can be averaged over all soft tissue of the body to give a representative mean value for whole-body composition. Mazess, Peppler, and Gibbons (1984) published results on 18 subjects assessed for total body composition by DPA and by underwater weighing and found that percent-fat estimates from the two methods were highly correlated (r = .87, SEE = 4.3%). Further they found that the difference between methods was closely related to the bone mineral content of the fat-free body (Mazess, Peppler, and Gibbons 1984).

The estimate of body composition from densitometers is derived from the relative attenuation of the photons in soft tissue (ST), which changes in proportion to the fat content as the dual energy radiation source scans over the soft tissue of the body. R_{ST} [153]Gd ranges from 1.32 for a 100% fat sample to 1.47 for a 100% lean sample, and a change of 0.01 R_{ST} corresponds to a 4% change in body fatness (Mazess et al., 1984). The precision of determining R_{ST} was initially found to be 0.005 g/cc, which is equivalent to 2% body fat. This precision has been reduced to 0.0023 g/cc in our laboratory, equivalent to a fat content of 1.1% for a sample of 104 adult women, using DER (Hansen et al., in press). With this excellent precision the method has great promise for determining the fat content of the soft tissue of the body.

Calibrating Assessment Methods

The calibration of DPA and DER was studied comparing the relation of R_{ST} to the composition of simulated fat and muscle (alcohol and water mixtures) standards (%Fat = −518 R_{ST} + 725; Mazess et al., 1990). A ground beef calibration was carried out by Heymsfield, Wang, Kehayias, and Pierson (1989), with the 10-kg beef samples ranging from 4% to 83% fat. The percent-fat equation found was % Fat = −499 R_{ST} + 732.6, with a correlation of .99. The theory and validation of the DPA approach to total body composition was further investigated by Wang, Heymsfield, Aulet, Thornton, and Pierson (1989) in a sample of 28 subjects, as well as by Heymsfield, Wang, Kehayias, and Pierson, (1989) in a smaller sample of 13 subjects.

Validation Studies

On the 13 subject studied by Heymsfield, Wang, Kehayias, and Pierson, (1989), percent fat from body density correlated .92 with percent fat from DPA with a SEE of 3.2%. Using the mean of four criterion methods (percent fat from densitometry, total body water, total body potassium, and neutron activation analysis) the correlation increased to .95, and the SEE was equal to 2.5%. This is one of the lowest prediction errors found between two methods. The work of Wang et al. (1989) has extended the validation to a large sample size (99 males, 187 females, between 19 and 94 years). Percent fat from densitometry in males averaged 21.3% (mean age 49.3 years) and 20.2% for DPA. The correlation was .87, and the SEE was 3.4% fat. For females, percent fat averaged 28.6% from densitometry and 30.7% from DPA, with a correlation between methods of .81 and a SEE of 4.8% fat (Table 3.1). In our work with a much more homogeneous sample of women (Hansen et al., in press), we found a much lower SEE using DEXA to estimate the percent fat in a premenopausal, inactive female sample.

Part of the expected difference between investigations was the different variation in the bone mineral content of the fat-free body. For the Wang et al. (1989) sample, the bone mineral content expressed as a percent of the fat-free body was 5.4% with a standard deviation of 0.9%. For males, 49%, and for females, 59%, of the variation between percent-fat estimates by underwater weighing and by DPA could

Table 3.1   Comparison of Hydrodensitometry With Dual Energy Absorptiometry in Two Female Samples

Item	Hansen et al. (in press) ($N = 100$)	Wang et al. (1989) ($N = 187$)
	$\bar{X} \pm S$	$\bar{X} \pm S$
Age, years	34.1 ± 3.0	49.7 ± 17.9
% Fat$_{DPA/DRA}$	29.7 ± 6.8	30.7 ± 8.3
% Fat$_D$	29.9 ± 5.8	28.6 ± 7.8
r	.91	.81
SEE, %	2.4	4.8

be accounted for by variation in the bone mineral content of the fat-free body, reducing the prediction errors from 3.4% in males and 4.8% in females to 2.4% and 3.1%, respectively. It would have been helpful to see if the water content of the fat-free body also accounted for some of the variation between methods; however, body water was not measured in this sample. Without body water estimates, the density of the fat-free body can only be estimated assuming water increases as bone mineral decreases, which may not be the case in the older subjects of this sample. Furthermore, the formula used by Wang et al. (1989) to calculate the density of the fat-free body (D_{LBM}) is incorrect for two reasons.

$$D_{LBM} = \frac{D_b - 0.9 \, (F_{DPA})}{(1 - F_{DPA}) \, wt}$$

First, body weight (wt) should not appear in the formula, and second, the formula is derived from an incorrect relationship between whole-body density and fat and fat-free body. From Wang et al. (1989), we have:

(1) $$D_b = \text{Fat \% (fd)} + LBM \% \, (L_{BMD})$$

(2) $$D_{LBM} = \frac{D_T - 0.9 \, (F_{DPA})}{0.1 - F_{DPA}},$$

where fat density is 0.9 g/cc, D_{LBM} is the unknown density of LBM, F_{DPA} is fat fraction by DPA, and D_b is body density from densitometry. The correct formulas with traditional symbols are these:

(3) $$\frac{1}{D_b} = \frac{f}{df} + \frac{1-f}{d_{FFB}},$$

(4) $$d_{FFB} = \frac{1 - F_{DPA}}{\dfrac{1}{D_B} - \dfrac{f_{DPA}}{0.9}}.$$

With these incorrect derivations of Wang et al. (1989), it was found that the calculated density of the fat-free body can account for 90% of the variation between methods for males and 98% of the variation for females, where f is the fraction of fat and d_f is 0.9 g/cc, d_{FFB} is the unknown density of the fat-free body, and D_b is body density (Wang et al., 1989). Such a high association came from use of the incorrect formula above with the numerator of both variables (ΔF vs. D_{LBM}) being highly correlated and mathematically almost identical. By varying the percent fat from body density from 28% to 33%, while holding percent fat from DPA constant and assuming that all the errors between methods are due to the density of the fat-free body varying from the reference value of 1.10 g/cc, it is possible to produce Table 3.2. From Table 3.2, it is clear that with a lower percent-fat estimate found from body density than from DPA, the fat-free body density must be greater than 1.10, not less than 1.10 as found from Wang et al. (1989).

Soft Tissue Versus Whole-Body Composition

Another problem with these comparisons of percent fat from body density and DPA is that the percent fat from DPA is of the soft tissue and not whole-body. It is therefore an overestimate of total body fatness, which can be estimated from DPA by converting soft tissue percent fat to a whole-body percent-fat basis for each subject. In the case of the female sample from Wang et al. (1989),

$$\text{fat}_w = \frac{fat_s\,(wt_s)}{wt} = \frac{0.307\,(51.2 - 2.4)}{51.2} = 29.3\%.$$

Thus, when soft-tissue percent fat is converted to whole-body percent fat, we have a 1.4% decrease. Assuming the actual fat-free body weight of 36.9 kg (28% fat), the bone mineral would be 1.98 kg (53.7 g bone mineral per kg FFB; Wang et al., 1989). Adding the nonosseous mineral to the 1.98 kg would yield 2.4 kg total mineral. Body weight was 51.2 kg in the sample studied. It is unclear from the procedures described by Heymsfield, Wang, Kehayias, and Pierson (1989) and Wang et al. (1989) if these corrections to whole-body composition were considered; however, they are essential whenever comparisons with densitometry are made.

Table 3.2   Recalculated Density of the Fat-Free Body Based on the Discrepancy Between DPA Percent Fat and Density Percent Fat

Variable	Recalculated body densities and different levels of discrepancy between DPA and D_b					
Body density g/cm^2	1.0356	1.0334	1.0312	1.0291	1.0270	1.0248
% Fat (D_b)	28.0	29.0	30.0	31.0	32.0	33.0
% Fat (DPA)	30.0	30.0	30.0	30.0	30.0	30.0
Theoretical fat-free D_b	1.107	1.1035	1.100	1.0965	1.0931	1.0896

Note. Calculations were derived using Wang et al. (1989) equation.

Mineral Content in Adult Females

A final problem with the results of Wang et al. (1989) that must be addressed relates to the density of the fat-free body in the young female adult samples and, in particular, the water and mineral contents. Assuming that the mineral content of reference man is 6.8%, which includes both osseous and nonosseous mineral and applies to the general population of young adult males, I estimated (Lohman, 1986) that the female adult population had a mineral content of 6.2% and a fat-free body density of 1.09 g/cc. (For the mineral content we used single photon absorptiometry on children and adults and did not have more direct estimates of total bone mineral; Lohman, Slaughter, et al., 1984). In the work of Wang et al. (1989), considerably lower bone mineral content was found for males than for females, 4.8% versus 5.4% of the fat-free body, in their heterogeneous sample of a wide age range. As shown in Table 3.3, in a study by Mazess et al. (1990) six males had a lower mineral content (5.4%) than females (6.1%). In Mazess et al. (1984) using DPA, the mean bone mineral content of the fat-free body in four young adult men was 6.9%, and for three females, 7.9%. In our work with young adult females using DEXA to estimate body composition and bone mineral content, we found a 7.2% mineral content of the fat-free body when we converted the osseous bone mineral content (2.56 g) to total mineral (3.11 g) and divided by a fat-free body mass (42.9 kg). To convert the estimates of Mazess et al. (1990) to total bone mineral content of the fat-free body, one must estimate the nonosseous mineral portion of the body and add it to the osseous mineral portion, because DER and DPA only estimate the mineral content from bone, leaving out the significant nonosseous fraction of the total mineral content of the body.

If we assume that a 17.6% proportion of all mineral in the body resides in the nonosseous compartment (Brozek et al., 1963), then the osseous bone mineral obtained from DER can be divided by 0.824 to derive an estimate of the total mineral content of the body. Thus, in the work of Mazess et al. (1990), 12 subjects had a bone mineral mass of 2.82 kg, or a total mineral mass of 3.42 kg. This calculates to 6.86% of the fat-free soft tissue mass. If we add the 3.42 kg of mineral to the 49.9 kg of fat-free soft tissue mass, we obtain an estimate of the fat-free body mass (53.3 kg). Dividing 3.42 by 53.3 gives a 6.4% mineral content of the fat-free body in this sample. Comparing results in the six males and six females, we again find males (6.1%) to have less mineral content in their fat-free body than females (6.7%, Table 3.3). Similar results are found in the Mazess et al. (1984) sample (Table 3.3). Thus, further work will be needed to sort out the fat-free body composition of young adult females, especially the mineral content and water content of the fat-free body, and obtain the proper alternative to the Siri formula based on the actual fat-free body density of young adult females.

The Need for DER Validation and Cross-Validation Studies

With the promising approach to total body composition by DER (Figure 3.2) there is a great need for careful validation and cross-validation studies with

Table 3.3   Estimation of Mineral Content of Fat-Free Body (FFB)

| Variable | Mazess et al. (1990) | | Mazess et al. (1984) | | Hansen et al. (1991) |
	Males (N=6)	Females (N=6)	Males (N=4)	Females (N=3)	Females (N=100)
Osseous bone mineral, g	3.20	2.39	3.49	2.84	2.56
Estimated total bone mineral, g	3.88	2.90	4.24	3.47	3.11
Fat-free soft tissue, kg	59.6	40.3	—	—	—
Fat-free body mass, kg	63.5	43.2	60.9	44.3	42.3
Mineral content of FFB, %	6.1	6.7	6.9	7.9	7.3

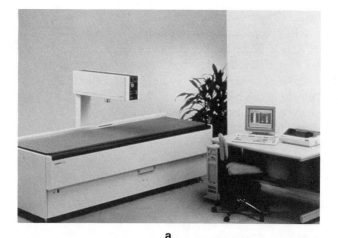

Figure 3.2   a. Dual energy X-ray absorptiometric equipment. b. Print-out of regional and total BMD from DEXA. *Note.* Photos courtesy of Lunar Corporation, Wisconsin.

laboratories working together to establish the advantages and limitations of the technology. Initial research into a new method often emphasizes the initial success of a given method, and it is only after several investigations have been conducted that some of the limitations emerge. To add to the complexity of validation studies and the introduction of soft-tissue composition rather than fat-free body composition, and bone mineral mass rather than total body mineral mass, for DER, three different technologies from three different companies are available to estimate body composition from X-ray exposure and analysis. The DER by Hologic (QDR-1000) uses an X-ray tube and an attending X-ray generator voltage and integrating detector and internal calibration wheel rather than a photon-counting detector. Software utilizing this new system for body composition assessment has only recently been developed, and major body composition studies have yet to be published from this new technology. The DER by Lunar Radiation (DPX) is an X-ray-based scanner that uses a filtered beam and an energy-discriminating photon-counting detector. Because the filter energies of the X ray are similar to those of Lunar's DPA system, they have utilized previous software from their DPA to obtain total body composition. The DER by Norland (XR26) uses two photon-counting detectors along with an X-ray tube and allows for beam intensity to vary with variation in patient thickness. By careful coordination among laboratories, comparisons can be made among instruments and technologies, among populations, and among other methodologies, enabling better estimates of the biological variation of the fat-free body composition to be separated out from technical variation. Some of this coordination may come about at a body composition standardization conference planned for 1993.

Regional Body Composition

One of the untapped potentials of DPA and DER is the estimation of regional body composition. Especially for the estimation of trunk composition and abdominal fat, this method may offer a practical way to validate anthropometric dimensions as indices of abdominal fat. Because of the association of visceral fat with risk of chronic diseases such as diabetes and coronary heart disease, the search for practical methods of assessing regional body composition is ongoing. In a recent paper by my colleagues (Going et al., 1990), the association of trunk soft tissue composition by DPA was examined in 82 young adult females. The test-retest reliability coefficient of the R_{ST} from a spine scan was found to be very high ($r = .97$). The soft tissue trunk attenuation coefficient (R_{ST}) was correlated most highly ($r = -.88$) with the sum of three skinfolds on the trunk (subscapular, abdomen, and superailiac), while body density was most highly correlated with the sum of four skinfolds, namely, triceps, subscapular, abdomen, and calf ($r = -.87$). The correlations of R_{ST} with BMI and D_b were $-.62$ and $.78$, respectively.

From these results we see that trunk subcutaneous fat relates more closely to the abdominal R_{ST} than to whole-body composition. It is likely, in those individuals for whom R_{ST} is overpredicted from the sum of three trunk skinfolds, that more abdominal visceral fat may be contributing to their total trunk fat. Studies with computer-assisted tomography and DER will help to validate this approach, which may turn out to be the most useful laboratory method for estimating trunk and abdominal visceral fat.

In addition to estimates of trunk composition, DPA and DER offer appendicular estimates of bone, lean, and fat composition. Recent work by Heymsfield et al. (1990) suggests that this approach could lead to an improved method for qualifying human skeletal muscle mass in limbs as well as in the total body.

Sources of Variation in DER and DPA

Body thickness, variation in fat distribution, and variation in the fat content of bone marrow are the major biological sources of variation affecting the accuracy of bone mineral estimates and fat content of the soft tissue from DRA and DPA. Hangartner and Johnston (1990) found that homogeneous layers of simulated fat (lucite) spread over a phantom had no influence on results as thickness level increased. There was an effect only if the fat thickness over the bone was increased (causing a reduction in bone mineral content) relative to the thickness over the soft tissue, or if the fat thickness over the bone was decreased (causing an increase in bone mineral content). This differential effect of fat distribution is a factor in bone estimates and in estimating the bone mineral content of the fat-free body; however, its contribution to error is probably small, because the amount of fat next to the bone is likely not very different from that over bone. A second aspect is the assumption that the soft-tissue composition over the regions of the body without bone (6,000 pixels) is similar to the soft-tissue composition over bone (5,000 pixels). Mazess et al. (1990) has estimated that the mass of soft tissue used for the estimate of body composition comprises about 55% to 60% of the total soft-tissue mass. Thus, by this method we are basing our estimates of whole-body composition on slightly more than one half of the desired body mass of interest. This assumption of uniformity of composition in the soft tissue not measured is likely the major source of error in the DRA and could lead to less accurate whole-body estimates if there is a systematic difference in the fat content of soft tissue in these two areas from individual to individual and from population to population.

In relation to the thickness of the body, Mazess has shown an increase in R_{ST} over the range of body thicknesses between 15 to 25 cm and has incorporated corrections for this effect by using subject thickness measurements in the calculations (Mazess et al., 1990). Subjects above 25 cm in thickness need further investigation, which has not yet been reported in the literature.

Variation in the fat content of bone marrow has also been shown to affect bone mineral estimates; however, this effect is thought to contribute only a small error to these estimates (Hangartner & Johnston, 1990). Variation in the fat content of bone marrow will not be detected by the soft-tissue R_{ST} and is thus a small source of additional variation in estimating total body fat content.

A final source of variation that needs to be discussed is the assumption that the lean content of the soft tissue has a constant density from individual to individual, so that the R_{ST} reflects variation in fat content and not variation in lean composition. Since variation in the hydration of fat-free body is largely a result of bone mineral content variability, this source of variation may not be significant in young adults except if a subject is measured in the dehydrated state. However, in children and the aged the water content of lean tissue may differ from young adults, and thus it is an additional source of error between populations that needs to be taken into account by future researchers.

Variation Between Densitometry and DER in a Homogeneous Population

Most studies to date using DPA and DER have used heterogeneous populations of subjects varying widely in age and weight. In contrast, the work in our laboratory has focused on a relatively homogeneous population under which the biological variation of the method can be more easily quantified. We found that the standard error of estimate for predicting % Fat $-$ D_b from percent fat from DEXA was 2.4% in a sample of 100 women between 28 and 39 years of age (Hansen et al., 1991). The prediction error for body density from percent fat from DEXA was 0.0053 g/cc and was lowered to 0.0040 g/cc when percent bone mineral content of the body was entered into the multiple regression equation. Taking away the technical error for measuring body density and variation associated with fluctuations in the water content (0.0030 g/cc; Jackson et al., 1988) leaves us with the remaining error of 0.0026 g/cc:

$$\sqrt{.(0.0040)^2 - (0.0030)^2} = \sqrt{0.000057} = 0.0026 \text{ g/cc.}$$

Thus, in this sample of inactive premenopausal women we have an estimate of the biological error estimating percent fat from DEXA. The error of 0.0026 g/cc corresponds to an error of 1.2% fat in this population.

Summary

Opportunity to determine the mineral content of the body with low radiation exposure and high precision as a function of age, gender, and activity level is one of the major areas to which DER will contribute in the coming years. Second, DER estimates of bone mineral may lead to improved estimates of the fat-free-body density in different populations from children to the elderly. In young adult female populations, further work is needed to determine that previous estimates of the water and mineral contents of young adult women (74% water and 6% mineral content of the fat-free body) are correct. Because of the high reliability with which estimates of fat content of the soft tissue can be obtained with DER, and because of initial results indicating its high validity in relation to body density, DER is presently being evaluated as an alternative criterion method to densitometry. In addition, DER offers the possibility of estimating regional composition and may enable indirect estimation of abdominal fat. With the different technologies emerging that utilize DER to estimate soft tissue for body composition as well as to assess bone mineral, there is a great need to conduct interinvestigator studies to compare technologies and remove systematic differences associated with methodological factors from biological variation. Furthermore, the limitations and assumptions of the DER approach need further evaluation so that standard error of estimate and prediction equations can be developed for various populations. In the coming years, much research will be accomplished in this area, leading to new understanding of biological variation in body composition and its implications for health.

Chapter 4

Prediction Equations and Skinfolds, Bioelectric Impedance, and Body Mass Index

How effective in predicting body composition are skinfold and bioelectric impedance equations as compared to body mass index? Are prediction equations population or investigator specific, and how can these equations be utilized in the field most effectively? What use, if any, can be made of body mass index as a predictor of body composition in future research studies?

The development of bioelectric impedance to assess body composition by measuring the resistance of the body to an electrical current has renewed the controversy over the effectiveness of various field measures for assessing body composition. In a letter to the editor, Mazess (1990) points out: "To ascertain the validity of BIA (bioelectric resistance), resistance (R) alone must be related to composition independent of height or weight" (p. 178). He goes on to say: "If BIA is valid then R alone should correlate highly with fat-free body mass, fat mass, and/or percent body fat. The prediction of fat mass or even fat-free mass, from R alone is better than the prediction from skinfold thicknesses or arm circumference" (p. 178). In contrast to Mazess's view is the viewpoint of Lukaski, who found that skinfolds predicted percent fat with a standard error of estimate of 3.9%, while resistance index (HT^2/R) and body weight predicted percent fat (from densitometry) with a SEE of 2.7% (Lukaski, Bolonchuk, Hall, & Siders, 1986). Adding to the controversy are the results of Jackson, Pollock, Graves, and Mahar (1988), who found no improvements in the prediction of percent fat or fat-free body using BIA as compared to body mass index (BMI). They conclude that skinfolds predict percent fat much better (SEE 3.4%) than either BIA (4.6%) or BMI (4.5%) and that, for BIA, height and weight are the major determinants of BIA prediction accuracy. Yet Graves, Pollock, Calvin, Van Loan, and Lohman (1989) found that when prediction equations developed on the same BIA instrument were cross-validated, they obtained a SEE similar to the original samples (3.5% fat from densitometry) and considerably lower than BMI. In the early work of Segal et al. (1985), large prediction errors (5% fat) were found from BIA and percent fat by densitometry; however, in a later study, Segal, Van Loan, Fitzgerald, Hodgeson, and Van Itallie (1988) found smaller prediction errors. Finally, in the recent work of Baumgartner, Chumlea, and Roche (1988), using bioelectric impedance phase angle (reactance over resistance), a higher correlation was found with percent fat from densitometry than for BMI or skinfolds when phase angle was measured on the trunk rather than whole-body.

In addressing the question of the effectiveness of BIA equations to predict body composition, we must first have a solid grasp of the literature on body mass index and of skinfold prediction equations. We also need to understand the theoretical aspects of the components of bioelectric impedance, namely, resistance (R), resistance index (Ht^2/R), reactance (Xc), phase angle (Xc/R), and impedance (Z). Let us start first with body mass index and its relation to body composition, then compare skinfolds with body mass index, and then proceed to bioelectric impedance and body composition, to gain a perspective on the literature. To fully appreciate the research conducted with BIA, one needs to be familiar with the work of many investigators and investigator teams. In particular, it is critical to address the Mazess (1990) concern related to the low association of R and body composition, which is universally acknowledged but interpreted differently among investigators.

Body Mass Index

In their article "Reassessment of Body Mass Index," Smalley, Knerr, Kendrick, Colliver, and Owen (1990) find a correlation between BMI and densitometry (% fat-D) of .82 in a sample of 213 women (% fat range 8.8 to 55.2, $\overline{X}$ = 26.3 ± 9.4) and .70 in 150 men (% fat range 5.0 to 52.9, $\overline{X}$= 20.9 ± 7.6). In both samples a wide age range (men, 18 to 82 years; women, 15 to 68 years) is present. The authors show that the major problem with body mass index is in the sensitivity of the index, as only 55.4% of women and 44.3% of men are diagnosed as obese by BMI if diagnosed obese by % fat-D.

Why is BMI limited in predicting percent fat for a given individual? First, it is obvious that the numerator, body weight, is influenced by the amount of muscle, organs, and skeleton as well as fat. Thus, an individual with a large musculoskeletal system in relation to height can have a BMI in the obese range and not be overfat. Similarly, individuals with a small skeletal frame or with a small musculoskeletal mass relative to their height will lead to an underestimate of their percent fat. Garn, Leonard, and Hawthorne (1986) have shown a correlation of .65 in men between percent lean body mass and BMI, indicating that BMI reflects the relative weight of both lean tissue and fat tissue. Slaughter and Lohman (1980) found that the SEE for predicting FFB from height in young men was larger (6.3 kg, CV = 9.8%) than in women (SEE = 3.5 kg, CV = 8.1%).

We can use these numbers to see how body mass index can change due to variation in FFB mass. Garn et al. (1986) have also shown that in children, adolescents, and adults, individuals with short legs for their height have higher BMI; thus this index reflects body proportions in addition to body composition. The small and negative association of BMI to stature in adults and positive association in children is similar to the association of stature with percent fat (Womersley & Durnin, 1977) and might not be a criticism of BMI as Garn et al. (1986) suggested.

In children we have a particularly difficult time interpreting BMI across age, as the musculoskeletal system is adding weight relative to height while fat development is also proceeding. The 50th percentile for BMI in males changes from 15.4 at 6 years of age to 21.5 in 17-year-olds, based on national norms established by the National Health Examination Survey (NHES), while the sum of two skinfolds (triceps plus subscapular) increases from 12 mm to 15 mm. (BMI and skinfolds at the 50th, 85th, and 95th percentiles are given in Appendix 4.1.) The results of Houtkooper, Lohman, Going, and Hall (1989) indicate that BMI can predict percent fat from density and water content with a SEE of 5.7%. Similarly, in the elderly, BMI can be a misleading index of fatness, because of differential rates of loss in muscle and bone mass among individuals.

Future Research With Body Mass Index

In his letter to the editor, McLaren (1987) states: "Only when BMI is abandoned in the study of obesity and more revealing and less misleading measurements are made, will we begin to understand the different forms of obesity" (p. 121). While I do not recommend total abandonment of this index in epidemiological, growth and development, and body composition studies, I do feel that research with BMI as the only measure of body composition in future studies will not contribute to new understanding. BMI needs to be included with skinfolds or bioelectric impedance and other laboratory body composition measures of muscle, bone, and fat (see chapter 5).

Smalley et al. (1990) state that the accuracy of the various height-weight indices for obesity has not been demonstrated, overlooking the work of Womersley and Durnin (1977), who compared all the major indices using height and weight as predictors of percent fat in the adult population. These indices include ratios of weight (W) to height (H), W to H^2 (Quetelet's index, or BMI), W to H^3, H to $W^{.33}$ (Sheldon's index), $W^{.33}$ to H (ponderal index), and percentage overweight based on sex, height, and age (W/DW), and all yielded results similar to those from body mass index (W/H^2) with all indices showing higher correlations in women than in men (see Table 4.1). Correlations are affected by the variability of the criterion variable in the sample (percent fat from densitometry); so it is better to compare SEEs within populations (men vs. women; Lohman, 1981). For the results found by Womersley and Durnin (1977), the SEEs within age group are somewhat smaller for women (5.4% fat) versus men (5.9% fat).

Table 4.1   Correlations of Indices of Height (H) and Weight (W) With Percent Fat From Densitometry

Indices	Mean correlation over five age groups	
	Men	Women
W/H	.55	.76
W/H^2	.55	.80
W/H^3	.51	.79
W$^{.33}$/H	.51	.79
H/W$^{.33}$	−.51	−.79
W/DW	.55	.79
Log of 4 skinfolds	.78	.82

Note. Calculations were derived using Womersley and Durnin (1977) equation.

Especially for women in the 30- to 39-year-old age group (SEE 3.9% fat), 40- to 49-year-old age group (SEE = 3.9% fat), and 50- to 68- year-old age group (SEE = 4.3% fat), the SEEs are somewhat less than for men (SEEs = 5.5% fat in these age groups). With higher correlations found by Womersley and Durnin (1977) for women (Table 4.1), one can ask why the SEEs are not lower yet than just indicated. The answer lies in the greater variability for women than for men found in the criterion percent fat. As an example, for women the mean and standard deviation in the 30- to 39-year-old group is 33.6 ± 8.7%. With a correlation of .90 between variables, the SEE can be calculated as

$$\text{SEE, } \% \text{ F} = 8.7 \sqrt{1.0 - (.9)^2} = 3.9\%.$$

For men 30 to 39 years of age, the mean and standard deviation for percent fat was 23.3 ± 6.7%. With a correlation of .56 between variables, the SEE is 5.6%.

Looking further at the SEEs, we can see that the ability of BMI to estimate percent fat is somewhat better within age groups than over a wide age range (Table 4.2). The Hansen et al. (in press) sample is not only a narrow age range but also contains only subjects with a sedentary physical activity level. In contrast to the conclusion drawn by Smalley et al. (1990) that BMI has a 95% confidence interval for predicting percent fat of 10% for women and 11% for men, we can see that the index may be somewhat improved within age group, rather than using one formula derived from all age groups, and that in women between 30 and 60 years of age the index is markedly better than in men. With this frame of reference we can go on to evaluation, skinfold equations, and BIA, asking whether these methods improve the SEEs of prediction over BMI.

Table 4.2   Standard Errors of Estimate for Prediction of Percent Fat by Densitometry

	% Fat (SEE) from BMI	
Wide age range	Men	Women
Womersley and Durnin (1977)	5.9	5.4
Smalley et al. (1990)	5.5	5.1
Jackson and Pollock (1985)	5.8	5.1
Narrow age range	Men	Women
Womersley and Durnin (1977)	5.1 (4.3 to 5.6)	4.8 (3.9 to 6.1)
Lohman et al. (1987)	4.7	4.5
Hansen et al. (in press)	—	3.5

Skinfold Prediction Equations Versus Body Mass Index

One of the most practical approaches to the assessment of body composition in the adult population ages 20 to 50 years of age is the use of skinfolds. Because 50% to 70% of body fat is located subcutaneously, selected skinfolds have been found to relate to overall body fatness (Lohman, 1981). The Jackson-Pollock skinfold equations, with the sum of three, four, or seven skinfolds and age used to estimate body density with percent fat calculated from body density, have been cross-validated for general use in the population (Jackson & Pollock, 1985). These skinfold equations were developed using a Lange skinfold caliper on a heterogeneous sample of subjects varying widely in percent fat. They appear especially useful for adults between 10% and 40% fat but may underestimate fatness in those over 40% fat. These equations were developed on large samples of white adults and cross-validated on additional samples (Jackson & Pollock, 1978; Jackson, Pollock, & Ward, 1980). In a summary of their work, Jackson and Pollock (1985) developed additional equations and tables for easy conversion of their skinfolds into body fatness as a function of age. Compared with BMI, Jackson and Pollock found considerably lower SEEs for their skinfold equations.

In addition to the Jackson-Pollock skinfold equations based on the sum of skinfolds (linear and quadratic polynomials for a curvilinear fit to body density) and age, Durnin and Womersley (1974) have used the log of the sum of four skinfolds (selected to represent trunk and limb fat) to predict body density in subjects from 17 to 72 years of age. They developed equations for five age groups and used the log of skinfolds to account for the nonlinear skinfold-density relationship; both Lange and Harpenden skinfold calipers were used on this sample of 209 men and 272 women. A comparison of the SEEs for predicting percent fat from skinfolds versus BMI with the Jackson-Pollock equations is shown in Table 4.3. It is clear that lower standard errors are found by Jackson and Pollock (1985) than by Durnin and Womersley (1974) for skinfolds and that

Table 4.3   Comparison of Standard Errors of Estimate (SEEs) Between Body Mass Index (BMI) and Skinfolds for Predicting Percent Fat From Densitometry

	SEE for % Fat-D	
Jackson and Pollock (1985)	Men	Women
BMI	5.8	5.1
Skinfolds	3.5	3.9
Durnin and Womersley (1974)	Men	Women
BMI	5.9	5.4
Skinfolds	4.6	4.9

BMI is much less effective, compared to skinfolds, in the Jackson-Pollock sample than in the Durnin-Womersley sample.

The controversy around BMI versus skinfolds and the discrepant prediction errors between investigations is characteristic of the field, with many researchers finding skinfolds considerably more effective than BMI and others finding skinfolds only somewhat better than BMI. The reasons for this difference may be associated in part with investigator differences in skinfold and body density measurement procedures and technical errors associated with these procedures.

Investigator Effects on Population-Specific Equations

There are two controversies with the use of these BMI and skinfold equations. One is the concept that skinfold equations are often population specific and inapplicable to other populations or even other samples of the same population. A second controversy relates to the accurate measurement of skinfolds and the various technical sources of error, including skinfold measurement technique, skinfold site location, skinfold caliper, and skinfold compressibility, which lead to prediction errors. In my review of this area (Lohman, 1981), I found that investigations designed to predict body fatness from skinfold varied in design, subject number and heterogeneity (homogeneous vs. varied, with respect to body fatness), skinfold sites measured, statistical analysis techniques, as well as technical description of skinfold sites. I pointed out, for example, that the suprailiac skinfold is defined differently by different investigators and that this must be taken into account in using a particular investigator's equations (Lohman, 1982).

A good example of investigator and investigation effects on skinfold measurements is the study that my colleagues and I conducted with four calipers and four investigators. For this study (Lohman, Pollock, Slaughter, Brandon, & Boileau, 1984) all four investigators were told to follow the same skinfold procedures but did not train together to see that they used the same measurement technique. Using one of the Durnin-Womersley equations (sum of triceps and subscapular) to determine the magnitude of methodological effects on percent-fat estimates, the mean fat content for this sample of 16 female college athletes ranged from 21.1 to 28.1 for the 16 combinations of caliper and investigator ($\overline{X}$ = 24.2 and S = 2.1). When the Jackson-Pollock equations (triceps, abdomen, suprailiac, and thigh) were used, the mean fat content was 20.3%, ranging from 16.8% to 25.6% over the 16 combinations. From this study, three important sources of variation emerged: (a) Mean fat content is affected by the equation selection—for instance, Durnin-Womersley gives higher percent fat than Jackson-Pollock; (b) the skinfold caliper used affects the mean fat content for a given equation (Table 4.4), with comparable results found using the Harpenden caliper and the Durnin-Womersley equations ($\overline{X}$ = 23.8% fat) as for using the Lange calipers with the Jackson-Pollock equation ($\overline{X}$ = 23.4% fat); and (c) the investigators obtained large systematic differences, especially at the suprailiac, abdomen, and thigh skinfold sites, and smaller differences for the triceps and subscapular sites. Difference among investigators also varied with caliper and skinfold site from 1 to 9 mm (Lohman, Pollock, et al., 1984). In an effort to minimize these sources of variation in future research, my colleagues and I organized a conference on the standardization of anthropometry, inviting investigators from the fields of exercise sciences, human biology, medicine, nutrition, and public health. The outcome of this conference was a standardization manual in which 47 anthropometric dimensions were given standardized definitions and descriptions (Lohman, Roche, & Martorell, 1988). An abridged version of this manual, providing only the descriptions and pictures of the standard anthropometric dimensions, has been recently published (Lohman, Roche, & Martorell, 1991).

Table 4.4 Differences Between Skinfold Calipers and Skinfold Equations in the Mean Sample Fat Content

Caliper	% Fat	
	Jackson-Pollock	Durnin-Womersley
Lange	23.4	26.9
Harpenden	19.6	23.8

Note. Calculations were derived using Lohman et al. (1984) equation.

Cross-Validation of Population-Specific Equations

With the important investigator sources of variation identified for skinfolds, it is critical to cross-validate regression equations developed by others on different populations and in different laboratories to determine their applicability. Age, gender, and ethnic group have all been identified as factors that affect fat distribution throughout the body, yielding different relationships between a given set of skinfolds and total body fatness. For example, if we adjust skinfolds in young and middle-aged men and women to the same body density, we find that women in both age groups have a lower amount of subcutaneous fat than men (Lohman, 1981). Thus, separate skinfold equations for women are different than for men, and this is well recognized in the field. The effects of age and ethnic group, however, are not well established, and this area remains one of the most important for investigations in the 1990s. Such equations specific to age group, gender, and ethnicity, including black, Hispanic, and Native American, as well as white, are needed to interpret the national probability skinfold data in terms of percent body fatness.

I described (Lohman, 1981) a procedure with seven principles for cross-validating such equations. To this list I would like to add an eighth and a ninth principle:

1. Report standard errors of estimate as well as correlation for each equation.
2. Compare predicted mean using new equation with actual mean using a criterion variable such as body density.
3. Fit curvilinear lines rather than assume linearity.
4. Calculate total error (E) as well as SEE.
5. Compare standard deviation of the predicted values with measured values.
6. Use large sample sizes.
7. Examine distribution of sample fatness if nonrandom sampling is used and note if sample is homogeneous (less than 5%) or heterogeneous (more than 7%) in fatness.
8. Don't publish a new equation on a new sample unless it can be shown to be a marked improvement over the many already published equations (i.e., the new equation has a lower SEE and a lower E and meets all criteria—1 through 7 above).
9. Change the intercept of an existing (previously published) equation if the total E is large, rather than develop a new equation (see Hansen et al., in press).

One way to utilize the present literature in developing generalized equations is to combine data rather than to continue to collect new data on new samples. The skinfold equation I developed (Lohman, 1981),

$$D = 1.0982 - 0.000815X + 0.00000084\ X^2$$
$$X = \text{sum of triceps, subscapular, and abdomen skinfolds,}$$

was based on the data of Sinning (1974) on 30 college wrestlers, Sloan (1967) on 50 college students, Lohman et al. (1978) on 61 college males, and Boileau et al. (1971) on 8 obese males using the sum of triceps, subscapular, and abdomen skinfolds. Curiously, this equation was found to cross-validate best on high school wrestlers and is being proposed for use as an index of minimal weight in the high school wrestling population. Results of cross-validation of this equation are presented in chapter 9. The research study of Segal et al. (1988) is also an example of combining data bases in an attempt to produce a more general equation for body composition estimation based on bioelectric impedance. The research of Gray, Bray, Gemayel, and Kaplan (1989) using Segal's equations on the obese is a model paper for extending present equations to new populations rather than developing new ones. The investigation by Teran et al. (1991) on 221 obese female adults shows the limitations of applying the Jackson-Pollock and Durnin-Womersly skinfold equations to this sample for subjects above 35% fat. It is unfortunate, however, that the new equation developed by these authors for the obese includes six circumferences and two skinfolds with no comparison of BMI, BIA, or skinfold equations with fewer sites than the eight dimensions given. Further, a comparison of circumferences versus skinfolds in the obese would help to establish whether circumferences are a better index than skinfolds and body mass index in this population, as has been suggested by some investigators.

Future Research With Skinfold Equations

Future research in skinfold equations needs to look at fat patterning differences with age, ethnic group, fatness level, and physical activity status. A change in fat patterning or distribution would change the skinfold-to-body-fat relationship, as we found in male children and youth with maturation (Slaughter et al., 1988). Because fat patterning on the trunk versus the limbs changes in prepubescent children to postpubescent adolescents, the equation for males changes in relation to the sum of triceps and subscapular skinfolds and percent fat.

In adults, with aging, the fat distribution may change (Lohman, 1981). At present, we cannot easily sort out the influences of changes in fat distribution with changes in density of fat-free body associated with bone mineral loss on body fatness prediction with age. For example, using the Jackson-Pollock equations on 30- and 50-year-old females with the sum of three skinfolds (triceps, abdomen, suprailiac) equal to 60 mm, we obtain a percent fat of 25.7% for the 18- to 22-year-old and 27% for the 55-year-old with the same skinfold. Is this change associated primarily with a change in fat distribution or with a change in the density of the fat-free body? All of the Durnin and Womersley (1974) equations, as well as the Jackson and Pollock (1985) equations, are based on the two-component model and assume constant density of the fat-free body with aging.

Bioelectric Impedance Versus Body Mass Index

In a study designed to compare the standard error of measurement for percent fat estimated by bioelectric impedance with those for skinfolds and densitometry, Jackson et al. (1988) measured 24 males and 44 females on two testers on 2 days for each of the three methods. The measurement error for whole-body resistance was 8.3 ohms in men and 13.9 ohms for women. This error was estimated to be equivalent to 1.4% fat for men and 1.5% fat for women. For skinfolds (sum of seven) and body density, the equivalent errors in terms of percent fat were about 1.0% for both methods in men and women. A significant amount of variation in both bioelectric impedance and body density was found with the subject and day interaction. The authors suggest that changes in body water over test days was the largest source of variation for these two methods. Coefficients of variation of 1.8% for men and 2.4% for women can be calculated from these bioelectric resistance measurements. Lukaski et al. (1986) found a CV of 2.0% for 14 men over 6 consecutive days. Over eight laboratories visited by two subjects, I found a CV of 2.8% in one subject and 2.1% on the other subject (Table 4.5). Van Loan and Mayclin (1987a) found a CV of 2.9% on nine subjects (2.4% on eight subjects, 6.9% on one subject) measured over 8 days. The data in Table 4.6 are given on a subject with a CV of 2.4% and one with a CV of 6.9%, to show the reader that a variation of almost 100 ohms is unusual (subject 3; Van Loan & Mayclin, 1987a) and may suggest that technical errors occurred in the instrumentation on Day 2 for Subject 3. A slightly larger CV (3% to 4%) was found by Roche (1985) in 11 women over 34- to 35-day periods, but no significant association was found with day of menstrual cycle.

Bioelectric Impedance as a Measure of Fat-Free Body Mass

Early research with bioelectric impedance by Segal et al. (1985) and Lukaski et al. (1986) established a relationship between FFB and resistive index or stature

Table 4.5   Daily Variation Within and Among Laboratories for Bioelectric Impedance

Source of variation	Resistance, ohms by day									
Intralaboratory[a]	CV	1	2	3	4	5	6	7	8	X	S
Subject 8	2.4%	521	521	534	509	534	524	550	538	529	12.4
Subject 3	6.9%	493	422	534	518	516	483	517	496	497	34.6

Interlaboratory	$\overline{X}^b$	S	CV	$\overline{X}^c$	S	CV
Subject 1	524	11	2.1	46.7	.98	2.1
Subject 2	389	11	2.8	73.4	2.26	3.1

Note. Calculations were derived using Van Loan & Mayclin (1987a) equations.
[a]($N = 8$ labs); [b]X, resistance, ohm; [c]$\overline{X}$, Ht^2/Resistance, cm^2/ohm.

Table 4.6   Prediction Error of Fat-Free Body Mass From Densitometry Using Bioelectric Impedance as Predictor

Investigator	SEE, kg
Lukaski et al. (1986)	
Men	2.5
Women	2.0
Lohman et al. (1987)	
Men	2.8
Women	2.1
Segal et al. (1988)[a]	
Men	2.9, 3.3, 3.6, 3.5
Women	2.1, 2.3, 2.4, 2.5

[a]SEE from four different samples.

square divided by resistance in ohms (L^2/R). The theoretical basis for this approach is reviewed by Lukaski (1987). The theory is that the volume of a conductor is related to the length (L) and its impedance (Z). Impedance of the body is affected by the specific resistivity and volume of the conductor. For the body the conductor of the electrical current is the fat-free body mass, or, more specifically, the total body water. It can be shown that the volume of the conductor (fat-free body) can be predicted as follows:

$$V = p \ (L^2/Z)$$

where p = specific resistivity of the fat-free body
L = length of the conductor
Z = impedance of the conductor.

It can be shown that impedance is the sum of resistance (R) plus reactance (Xc) of the body as follows:

$$Z = \sqrt{R^2 + X_c^2}$$

and since Xc is much smaller than R,

$$Z \sim R.$$

Thus

$$V = p \ (L^2/R).$$

Thus, when body density has been used as a criterion variable, FFB and percent fat have been calculated, and resistive index (L^2/R) and weight or resistance (R), weight and height squared have been used as the predictors. The SEEs range from a low of 2.0 kg (Lukaski et al., 1986) to a high of 5.1 kg (Jackson et al., 1988). Given that body water can be predicted with a SEE between 1.5 kg and 2.1 kg from BIA and that the water content of the fat-free body is 73%, we would expect errors of 2.1 kg to 2.9 kg for FFB mass from bioelectric impedance.

Three major studies substantiate the findings, as summarized in Table 4.6. In a follow-up study by Graves et al. (1989) using a different sample of subjects and the interuniversity protocol (Lohman et al., 1987), the authors developed a prediction equation with a SEE, much lower than that of their previous work (Jackson et al. 1988), of 2.6 kg, using L^2/R and body weight. The cause of the discrepancy between investigations in unknown, but I suspect the presence of a few outlines in the Jackson et al. (1988) sample originating in faulty resistance values from poor electric contact or from instrument instability such as indicated in the Van Loan reliability data on Subject 3 (Table 4.5).

The equations of Kushner and Schoeller (1986) and Lukaski et al. (1986) are characterized by large regression coefficients for L^2/R and small coefficients for weight. Davies, Jagger, and Reilly (1990), using $H_2^{18}O$ to estimate body water, also find low coefficients for weight and high coefficients for (L^2/R) (see Table 4.7). Similar results are found for total body water estimates from bioelectric impedance in patients with chronic obstructive pulmonary disease (Schols, Wouters, Soeters, & Westerterp, 1991). The work of Van Loan and Mayclin (1987a), Van Loan, Boileau, Christ, et al. (1990), and Segal et al. (1985) has shown larger prediction errors for estimating total body water and regression equations with larger coefficients for body weight. The investigations mentioned in Table 4.7 all have in common the use of mass spectroscopy to determine total body water, with one exception. In contrast to the results in Table 4.7 are results from the interinvestigator study of the six laboratories preivously mentioned, where three laboratories also measured total body water using deuterium dilution by infrared spectrophotometry, and the results of densitometry and hydrometry were presented in this subsample (Van Loan, Boileau, Christ, et al., 1990). In this study FFB could be predicted with a lower SEE from densitometry (SEE =

Table 4.7   Total Body Water Equations from Bioelectric Impedance With Low Regression Coefficients for Body Weight

Investigator	L^2/R	WT	Intercept	SEE
Kushner and	.396 ♂	.143	8.4	1.7
Schoeller (1986)	.386 ♀	.105		0.9
Davies et al. (1990)	.38	.18	4.7	1.5
Schols et al. (1991)	.44	.13	3.3	1.8

2.6 kg) than from body water (SEE = 3.2 kg), opposite to hypothesis, namely, that body water is a better representative of body conduction than fat-free body mass, which includes bone. I suspect that intra- and interlaboratory technical errors in estimation of body water among the three laboratories are a major reason why larger SEEs were found when body water was used as the criterion variable. The prediction equations were similar between the two methods (water vs. density) except for males, where fat-free body was estimated from total body water (TBW). The equation,

$$FFB_{TBW} = 0.39 \, L^2/R + 0.54 \, wt - .06 \quad SEE = 3.7 \text{ kg,}$$

with its high SEE (3.7 kg) and low regression coefficient for (L^2/R) (0.39) as compared to body weight (0.54), further suggests that this criterion variable (body water) is not working as well as it might if it were measured more accurately. In contrast, fat-free body from densitometry (FFB_d) in males was predicted much better in this sample:

$$FFB_d = 0.50 \, L^2/R + 0.36 \, wt + 2.9 \quad SEE = 3.0 \text{ kg.}$$

A critical study to help resolve the prediction accuracy of total body water and fat-free body mass would be to have different laboratories measure the same subjects for body water after each had been measured by whole-body impedance. This experimental design would help to address the issue of investigator-specific errors versus population-specific errors. For example, the work of Kushner and Schoeller (1986) demonstrated the lowest SEE for predicting body water (SEE = 0.9 to 1.7 kg). When the equations were cross-validated on an Arizona sample of older men, body water was predicted within a SEE of 2.4 liters (l) and, for an Illinois sample of older men, 3.2 l (Going, Hewitt, Williams, Lohman, & Boileau, in press). For females the SEEs were 1.5 l (AZ) versus 1.8 l (IL) as compared to a SEE of 0.9 l (Kushner & Schoeller, 1986). If these independent samples were all measured by the three laboratories (Schoeller, Lohman, & Boileau,), and samples were sent for body water assessment to all three laboratories, we could determine the investigator contribution to the measurement error. Until these interlaboratory comparisons are conducted, we are left with large differences among laboratory prediction errors that cannot easily be explained by sampling variation.

Interlaboratory Equations: Two Approaches

Earlier in this chapter I cited the interinvestigator study of Segal et al. (1988) as an example of one excellent way to develop generalized and prediction equations for body composition assessment. Data from four laboratories were combined into one analysis to predict fat-free body mass from multiple regression equations using resistance, stature squared, and body weight on 1,069 men and 498 women between the ages of 17 and 62 years. Data were analyzed by laboratory, gender and fatness category, and equations were proposed for men under and over 20% fat and for women under and over 30% fat. In a critical follow-up study by Gray et al. (1989), the cross-validation of these equations by Segal et al. (1988) was conducted. Gray and co-workers found that the equations of Segal overpredicted FFB by 2.5 kg (underestimated fatness) in subjects between 41% and 48% fat and by 4 kg to 5 kg in subjects between 48% and 59% fat. For subjects between 9% and 41% fat, the Segal equation overpredicted FFB by about 1 kg. Gray et al. (1989) presented a new equation for women over 48% fat as well as equations for women and men in general. Characteristic of Gray's equations and the Segal et al. (1988) equations for Laboratory A for women and Laboratory B for men are larger effects of resistance (larger regression coefficients) and small effects of body weight (small regression coefficients).

Comparing Equations Among Laboratories

Variation in the regression coefficients among laboratories for resistance and weight is the major limitation of the combined equation of Segal et al. (1988), which includes results from some laboratories where resistance was contributing very little to the prediction of FFB (low regression coefficients) (Table 4.8). To illustrate this effect, let us compare results of Labs A and B for men from a hypothetical individual weighing 70 kg and with a stature of 170 cm, a resistance of 470 ohms, and an age of 30 years.

According to Lab A,

$$\begin{aligned} FFB &= 0.00109 \; ht^2 - 0.0161R + 0.410wt - 0.154 \; age + 8.1 \\ &= 31.5 - 7.57 + 28.7 - 4.62 + 8.1 \\ &= 56.1 \text{ kg or } 19.8\% \text{ fat.} \end{aligned}$$

Table 4.8   Interlaboratory Investigation by Segal et al. (1988) and Gray et al. (1989)

Sample	Regression equations
Women > 48% (Gray)	FFB, kg = $0.000985 \; ht^2 - 0.0387R + 0.158 \; wt - 0.124 \; age + 29.6$
Women > 30% (Segal)	FFB = $0.000912 \; ht^2 - 0.0147R + 0.299 \; (wt) - 0.070 \; age + 9.4$
Women < 30% (Segal)	FFB = $0.000646 \; ht^2 - 0.0140R + 0.421 \; (wt) + 10.4$
Lab C (Segal)	FFB = $0.000942 \; ht^2 - 0.0141R + 0.311 \; (wt) - 0.145 \; age + 10.9$
Lab A (Segal)	FFB = $0.00112 \; ht^2 - 0.0380R + 0.211 \; (wt) - 0.130 \; age + 27.2$
Women (Gray)	FFB = $0.00151 \; ht^2 - 0.0344R + 0.140 \; (wt) - 0.158 \; age + 20.4$
Men > 20% (Segal)	FFB = $0.000664 \; ht^2 - 0.0212R + 0.628 \; (wt) - 0.124 \; age + 9.3$
Men < 20% (Segal)	FFB = $0.000886 \; ht^2 - 0.0300R + 0.427 \; (wt) - 0.070 \; age + 14.5$
Lab A (Segal)	FFB = $0.00109 \; ht^2 - 0.0161R + 0.410 \; (wt) - 0.154 \; age + 8.1$
Lab B (Segal)	FFB = $0.00124 \; ht^2 - 0.0663R + 0.263 \; (wt) - 0.228 \; age + 41.35$
Men (Gray)	FFB = $0.00139 \; ht^2 - 0.0801R + 0.187 \; (wt) + 39.83$

If we change resistance by 40 ohms (430 ohms), we will change the estimated fat content only 1%.

$$FFB = 56.7 \text{ kg or } 18.9\% \text{ fat}$$

According to Lab B,

$$FFB = 0.00124 \ ht^2 - 0.0663 \ R + 0.263 \ wt - 0.228 \ age + 41.35$$
$$= 35.84 - 31.16 + 18.41 - 6.84 + 41.35$$
$$= 57.6 \text{ kg or } 17.7\%.$$

If we change resistance to 430 ohms, we will change the estimated fat content by 3.8%, or almost 4 times the effect. We can see by this example the large difference between investigators in the association of resistance and body composition, with a 40-ohm change corresponding to a 1% to 4% variation in fat content.

Let us compare these equations with those using resistance index (L^2/R) and weight as the predictors, using an equation of Lukaski et al. (1986):

$$FFB = 0.756 \ (L^2/R) + 0.110 \ wt + 0.107 \ X_c - 5.46$$
$$= 0.756 \ (61.49) + 0.110(70) + 0.107 \ (60) - 5.46$$
$$= 46.49 + 7.7 + 6.4 - 5.46$$
$$= 55.13 \text{ kg or } 21.2\% \text{ fat}.$$

Changing the resistance to 430 ohms, FFB = 59.45 kg or 15.1% fat, or a 6.1% change in fat content.

Valhalla Interuniversity Study

To try to better understand this interinvestigator difference, I obtained the cooperation of laboratory investigators (Wilmore, Boileau, Sinning, Van Loan, Golding, Heymsfield, Pollock) and a cross-validation sample (Pollock & Graves), and Valhalla Scientific offered to provide each laboratory with a bioelectric impedance analyzer and funding for each laboratory to standardize all measurements prior to the study. In a unique departure from past research, all laboratories followed one set of standardized procedures for body density, skinfolds, and bioelectric impedance assessment. The results for each laboratory are given in Table 4.9. From these results it is clear that the SEEs, which vary from 2.3 kg to 2.8 kg FFM, are somewhat, but not a great deal, higher than the 2.1 kg found by Lukaski et al. (1986) in a combined sample of men and women.

If we compare the two extreme laboratories (A and D) among all six for regression coefficients, we find the following changes in our hypothetical subject for a change from 470 to 430 ohms (Table 4.10). For Lab A, a 2.7% change in body fatness is predicted from a 40-ohm resistance change; for Lab D, a 5.0% change.

Table 4.9   Interlaboratory Investigation Regression Equations Among Laboratories for Prediction of FFB, kg

Laboratory	Equation	SEE, kg	R^2
A	$Y = 0.34\ L^2/R + 0.41$ wt $+ 2.4G + 8.2$	2.5	94.7
B	$Y = 0.50\ L^2/R + 0.28$ wt $+ 1.7G + 7.1$	2.6	93.3
C	$Y = 0.44\ L^2/R + 0.31$ wt $+ 2.1G + 8.9$	2.3	96.4
D	$Y = 0.61\ L^2/R + 0.25$ wt $+ 1.2G + 2.7$	2.4	96.7
E	$Y = 0.40\ L^2/R + 0.37$ wt $+ 2.1G + 7.1$	2.7	95.7
F	$Y = 0.60\ L^2/R + 0.25$ wt $+ 0.8G + 3.4$	2.3	96.8

Combined equations: Male ($N = 153$); SEE = 2.9; FFB, kg $= 0.485\ L^2/R + 0.338$ wt $+ 5.32$

Female ($N = 153$); SEE = 2.1; FFB, kg $= 0.475\ L^2/R = 0.295$ wt $+ 5.49$; G = gender with $+1$ for male and -1 for female

Table 4.10   Percent Fat Change for a 40-Ohm Change in Resistance Based on Equations in Table 4.9

Laboratory	470 ohms	430 ohms
A	20.8	18.1
B	20.4	16.3
C	20.6	17.0
D	19.3	14.3
E	20.7	17.5
F	18.6	13.7

The most impressive aspect of the results summarized in Table 4.10 is the consistency with which the mean percent fat is obtained across laboratories for a hypotehtical 70-kg male with a 470-ohm resistance and 170-cm stature (20.8% to 18.6% fat). The predicted fat-free body mass using from 470 ohms for each labs varies from 57.0 kg to 55.4 kg. This close compatibility is part of the answer to the question raised by Deurenberg, Weststrate, Hautvast, and van der Kooy (1991), where FFB ranges from 50.3 kg to 55.3 kg, using different equations in the literature.

If we combine all six laboratories into one sample, we can compare BMI, skinfolds, circumferences, and bioelectric impedance to determine their comparative prediction accuracy, compared to densitometry, in the young adult. We found that skinfolds and bioelectric impedance are substantially better than circumferences and body mass index in this population and that skinfolds and impedance yield comparable results in both men and women (Table 4.11).

Table 4.11   Standard Error of Prediction of FFB and Percent Fat From the Combined Sample of Six Laboratories in Young Adult Males and Females

Prediction variables	Men (N = 153)		Women (N = 153)	
	FFB, kg (65.1 ± 8.0)	% Fat (14.2 ± 5.4)	FFB, kg (45.0 ± 5.2)	% Fat (23.1 ± 5.4)
Weight	4.1	5.1	2.9	4.8
Weight, ht	3.8	4.7	2.7	4.6
Wt/ht^2	6.4	4.7	4.4	4.5
L^2/R, wt	2.9	3.7 —	2.1	3.5 —
Skinfolds, wt	2.6	3.5 —	2.3	3.8 —
Circumference, wt	2.9	3.6	2.5	4.3

The equation that comes from the interuniversity study suffers from one limitation. The regression coefficients for L^2/R and weight are not sufficiently different from each other to yield good predictions for very lean and very fat subjects. Thus, use of this equation on athletes will overestimate their fatness, and in the obese, it will underestimate their fatness. This is shown by the cross-validation study of Graves et al. (1989), who show a smaller standard deviation for predicted percent fat, using the interlaboratory equation presented in Table 4.9, than that of Lukaski et al. (1986). This problem was further examined by myself and colleagues, correlating the residual error with percent fat and finding signficant association between the magnitude of error and the level of fatness (Lohman, Going, Hewitt, & Williams, 1990), as found by others (Segal et al., 1988). Thus, in a lean or athletic female sample we found the following equation (Houtkooper, Going et al., 1989)

$$FFB = 0.73 \ (L^2/R) + 0.16 \ wt + 2.0$$
$$[FFB = 0.73 \ (L^2/R) + 0.23 \ X_c + 0.16 \ wt + 2.0]$$

to apply better than our interuniversity equation:

$$FFB = 0.475 \ (L^2/R) + 0.295 \ wt + 5.49.$$

For young adult women between 20% and 30% fat, the above equation should work well but needs to be replaced by one with higher coefficients for L^2/R and lower ones for weight.

For women between 30% and 45% fat and above 45% fat, the formulas of Graves et al. (1989) are good candidates for cross-validation:

$$FFB \ (30\% \ to \ 45\%) = 0.00151 \ ht^2 - 0.0344 \ R$$
$$+ 0.140 \ wt - 0.158 \ age + 20.39.$$

$$FFB \ (>45\%) = 0.000985 \ (ht^2) - 0.0387 \ R + 0.158 \ (wt) - 0.124 \ age + 29.61.$$

Solving the Differences Between BMI and Skinfolds

In general, there is widespread appreciation by most investigators for the limited predictability of body composition from body mass index, and two major studies in this area were carefully reviewed earlier in this chapter. The question is, how much better are skinfold equations and bioelectric impedance equations than body mass index? From the viewpoint of Lukaski et al. (1986) and Kushner and Schoeller (1986), bioelectric impedance is considerably better than anthropometry and body mass index in estimating body composition. Furthermore, according to the recent results of Kushner et al. (1990), BIA can predict changes in fat-free mass in subjects undergoing weight loss with greater accuracy and precision than anthropometry.

Three large interlaboratory studies (Segal et al., 1988; Lohman et al., 1987; and Van Loan, Boileau, Christ, et al., 1990) found larger SEEs than that found by Lukaski and Kushner, and these authors conclude that bioelectric impedance is comparable to anthropometry and better than BMI. A careful analysis of variation in the regression equations among laboratories shows that the regression coefficient for L^2/R and for body weight varies considerably, so that a 40-ohm change in resistance corresponds to as much as a 6% change in body fatness by some equations and to change as small as 1% using other equations. This variation, which characterizes the state of the field, addresses Mazess's point (1990): To ascertain the validity of BIA, resistance alone must be related to composition, independently of height and weight.

In the equations by several authors predicting FFB or TBW from bioelectric impedance, we see a number of investigations where the predominant effect is with L^2/R rather than body weight. In investigations where the regression coefficients are higher for body weight, I believe these results are due not necessarily to the failure of the impedance-to-body-composition relationship but rather to the presence of investigator-specific factors related to measurement precision, instrument stability, and variation in protocol followed by each subject.

The second aspect of Mazess's (1990) statement—"If BIA is valid, then R alone should correlate highly with fat-free mass, fat mass and/or percent fat"—reflects a lack of awareness, fairly common in the field, of the theoretical aspects of conductivity. The resistance of the body to an electrical current is dependent on specific resistivity and volume of the conductor (fat-free body as the conductor, not fat). Thus R alone is not directly related to fat or fat-free body unless all subjects are similar in stature. This has recently been shown by Deurenberg et al. (1991), who found correlations of .85 and .77 with L^2/impedance and FFB in men and women and correlations of $-.48$ and $-.56$ with impedance (ignoring conductor length) and FFB (impedance and resistance are closely related). Thus, it is essential in the evaluation of bioelectric impedance to use the approaches of Lukaski, where L^2/R and body weight are predictors, or Segal, where L^2, R, and weight are predictors, and examine the magnitude of the regression coefficients with all variables in the equation.

Are skinfold equations better than body mass index? Most investigators indicate that skinfold equations are considerably better than BMI. In the work of Womersley and Durnin (1977), the improvement is especially apparent in men but not as much as in women, where BMI does better than in other populations. The rationale for this is shown in the research of Slaughter and Lohman (1980) where FFB in relation to body height is less variable than in men. For Jackson and Pollock (1985) and Jackson et al. (1988), skinfolds predict percent fat with much lower SEEs than does BMI. What can go wrong with the general use of skinfolds? Like bioelectric impedance, skinfold equations vary with investigator and can lead to systematic errors if the equation does not apply to the sample under investigation or if the investigator uses a measurement procedure or caliper for the skinfold sites that is different from that of the original investigation.

The solution to the dilemma at hand is to foster more interlaboratory investigations so that we can separate out investigator- from population-specific factors. A second solution is for all body composition investigations to include BMI, BIA, and skinfolds in their protocols, so that direct comparisons can be made. A third solution is to continue to standardize measurement procedures across laboratories. The measurement of body water content especially needs standardization in this area. A fourth solution is to follow the recent suggestion of Schoeller and Kushner (1991): "It is more important to turn our collective attention to cross-validating these equations [equations already published] and eliminating the least accurate and precise than in developing new equations" (p. 180).

Summary

In this chapter we have reviewed the research in the past 20 years on the question of prediction equations and prediction errors in estimating body composition from body mass index, skinfolds, and bioelectric impedance. Our focus has been on the size and stability of prediction errors and on the development of generalized prediction equations from each method. For all three approaches we have shown that there are population differences in equations, and thus there is a great need to develop equations specific to given populations, especially for BIA and skinfolds. In chapter 10 one such effort is reviewed in detail—the development of skinfold equations for the high school wrestling population. Equations within age, gender, ethnic group, physical activity, and various patient populations need to be developed and cross-validated.

APPENDIX 4.1

Body Mass Index (BMI) and Sum of Two Skinfolds by Age and Gender for Selected Percentiles

Age, years	BMI						Sum of two skinfolds					
	50th		85th		95th		50th		85th		95th	
	M	F	M	F	M	F	M	F	M	F	M	F
6	15.4	15.2	16.8	17.1	18.2	18.5	12	14	16	19	20	27
7	15.6	15.4	17.1	17.6	18.9	19.6	12	15	17	22	24	28
8	16.0	15.9	18.1	18.6	20.2	21.1	13	16	19	25	28	36
9	16.2	16.3	19.0	19.5	22.4	22.9	14	17	23	29	34	41
10	16.5	16.9	19.2	20.6	21.8	23.6	14	18	24	32	33	43
11	17.2	17.5	20.9	21.7	24.2	24.8	15	19	28	31	39	43
12	17.8	18.6	21.4	22.6	24.1	26.2	15	20	24	34	44	47
13	18.7	19.4	22.6	23.4	26.6	26.8	15	21	28	39	46	52
14	19.6	20.2	23.2	24.1	26.7	26.5	14	24	27	37	39	53
15	20.4	20.7	24.0	24.7	27.8	29.4	14	25	25	41	40	56
16	20.8	20.9	24.0	24.9	26.9	29.6	14	26	24	42	39	58
17	21.5	21.0	24.9	24.3	28.5	29.3	15	27	26	42	41	59

Note. Calculations were derived using NHES norms (1963-1968).

Chapter 5

Assessing Fat Distribution

Part of the failure of skinfold thicknesses to be perfect predictors of body fatness is related to the fact that in addition to the outside layer of subcutaneous fat sampled by skinfolds are the other depots of fat storage in the body: intermuscular fat, intramuscular fat, and internal fat found in the thoracic and abdominal cavities lining the vital organs. To what extent do individuals differ in their distribution of fat among the four depots, and what are the health consequences of this variation?

One of the most common methods of assessing body composition, namely, skinfold thicknesses, samples only one of the four major fat depots in the body, the subcutaneous fat. In addition, there are three other fat depots in the body—intermuscular fat, intramuscular fat, and fat in the abdominal and thoracic cavities. In recent years the association of central, upper body, and abdominal fat with increased risk of several chronic diseases has renewed interest in fat distribution throughout the body and in assessing total body fatness. This chapter explores the various approaches to the study of fat distribution and its relation to health and disease. Research is needed to compare various approaches of assessing variations in fat distribution and their independent effects on health. Because investigators have used different indices to assess fat distribution, and because different data analysis procedures have been used to determine the variation in fat distribution and its association with disease, no consensus has been reached on the best approach to assessing fat distribution in relation to health and disease.

The Four Major Fat Depots

In 1981 I presented estimates of the fat distribution in reference man and reference woman (Table 5.1) in relation to the four fat depots in the body. The inter- and intramuscular fat depots are small and most difficult to assess. Little research has been conducted to determine their variability or significance to health, and much of this chapter will therefore focus on subcutaneous fat and visceral fat in the thoracic and abdominal cavities.

Table 5.1   Fat Distribution in Reference Man and Woman

Fat location	Reference man	Reference woman
Essential fat (lipids of the bone marrow, central nervous system, mammary glands, and other organs), kg	2.1	4.9
Storage fat (depot), kg	8.2	10.4
Subcutaneous	3.1	5.1
Intermuscular	3.3	3.5
Intramuscular	0.8	0.6
Others (fat of thoracic and abdominal cavity), kg	1.0	1.2
Total fat, kg	10.3	15.3
Body weight, kg	70.0	56.8
% Fat	14.7	26.9

Note. Reprinted from *Human Biology,* Vol. 53, no. 2, pp. 181-225, by permission of the Wayne State University Press.

Central Versus Peripheral Fat

One approach to the assessment of fat distribution is to distinguish between central and peripheral fat, using various skinfold sites. This approach studies only one of the four major fat depots, namely, the subcutaneous fat, and uses skinfolds to assess variation among individuals. Garn, Sullivan, and Hawthorne (1988a) argue that four skinfolds found at the periphery and central locations (triceps, subscapular, iliac, and abdominal) are highly intercorrelated with their sum. Also, all four sites were not differentially related by decile to changes in blood pressure and serum cholesterol. Finally, factor analysis shows that the first factor is generalized fatness, accounting for most of the variance in skinfold thickness throughout the body (Garn, Sullivan, & Hawthorne, 1988b; Jackson & Pollock, 1976). Contrary to Garn et al. (1988a), Mueller and Wohlleb (1981) found the first and second principal components of skinfold variation in 44 samples to represent (a) index of fatness and (b) index of trunk extremity or proximal distal, regardless of sex, number of skinfold sites, measurement technique, or ethnicity. In their letter to the editor responding to Garn et al. (1988a), they argue that the data of Garn et al. (1988a) also show extremity fat having lower correlations with central fat than with other extremity sites and that if Garn et al. had looked at the partial correlation of tricep skinfolds with the risk variables, holding constant abdominal skinfolds, they would likely have found functional differences between central and peripheral fat (Mueller & Emerson, 1988). Garn et al. (1988b) reply that they have been studying fat distribution for 30 years apart from overall body fatness and feel that the association between individual skinfold site and total fatness is so close that there is little need to debate the location of a skinfold site, as fat distribution contributes only a small amount to the variation in skinfold thicknesses.

Baumgartner et al. (1986), using principal components, found that the trunk-extremity dimension accounts for between one third to one half of the total variation in fat patterning after the effects of total body fatness have been controlled. Another study on central versus peripheral fatness used principal components, with five skinfolds in adolescent obese and nonobese populations, and also removed overall body fatness from the data by dividing each skinfold site by the sum of the five skinfolds (Hattori, Becque, Katch, Rocchini, Boileau, et al., 1987). (The authors also used the approach of Healy and Tanner, 1981, using residuals from regression of the log of individual sites with the log of the sum of skinfolds, and found similar results.) Two major extracted components were found, with trunk versus extremity accounting for 60% of the variance and with upper versus lower trunk representing 20% of the common variance. They concluded that obese males and females had more fat in the trunk versus extremity than nonobese, and that obese males had more trunk fat at the lower skinfold sites, whereas obese females had more fat in the upper trunk in the adolescent sample. Because of their method of analysis, namely, removing variation in total fatness before data analysis, we cannot clearly see the magnitude of fat distribution differences in comparison with total body fatness, and thus it may be that the differences found are quite small relative to interindividual differences in total body fatness (Garn viewpoint) or large enough to have important functional value (Mueller viewpoint).

Closely related to the central versus peripheral skinfold distribution is the concept of fat patterning, which examines variation in skinfold thicknesses throughout the body as a function of age, gender, ethnic group, and genetics. Many studies show variation in fat patterning in different populations (e.g., Garn, 1955; Deutsch, & Mueller, 1985; Frisancho & Flegel, 1982).

Upper Versus Lower Trunk Fatness

A further delineation of fat distribution, or fat topography, comes from the observation that individuals differ in their fatness in the upper trunk versus the lower trunk as estimated by the waist-to-hip circumference ratio and its relation to cardiovascular disease (Larsson et al., 1984). In a large sample of middle-aged men this prospective study found significant association of coronary heart disease with waist-to-hip ratio (waist measured at the level of the umbilicus, and hip measured at the level of the iliac crest) as compared to body mass index, skinfolds, or circumferences by themselves. In a second prospective study, Lapidus et al. (1984) found the ratio of waist to hip (waist measured midway between lower rib margin and iliac crest, and hip measured at the widest point between hip and buttock) measured in women was a stronger predictor of cardiovascular disease than body mass index or subscapular and triceps skinfolds.

The construct here, in the ratio of waist-to-hip circumference, is the distinguishing between fatness in the lower trunk (i.e., hip and buttocks) versus fatness in the upper trunk (i.e. waist and abdomen areas). The fat depots assessed by this ratio are largely the subcutaneous and visceral, with subcutaneous fat being found largely in the lower trunk and subcutaneous and visceral fat both being measured in the waist circumference. Different waist and hip circumferences have been defined in the epidemiological studies, so that circumference location as well as fat depots are confounded in the ratio (see Lohman et al., 1988, for standardized sites suggested for future use). Since males are more likely to have upper trunk fatness (higher waist to hip ratio), and females, lower trunk fatness (lower waist to hip ratio), the terms *android obesity* and *gynoid obesity* are used to characterize these types of fat distribution.

Visceral Fat Distribution

Internal fat found in the thoracic and abdominal cavities of the body is not assessed by skinfolds and may vary in relation to subcutaneous fat. Visceral fat, often reflected in large waist and abdominal circumferences, is that portion of the internal fat in the abdominal cavity lining the intestinal tract. It has been hypothesized that visceral fat, rather than abdominal subcutaneous fat, is related to increased risk of chronic diseases and that the association of waist-to-hip ratio and disease is related to the amount of internal abdominal fat. Because abdominal fat can be measured only by computed tomography (CT) or magnetic resonance imaging (MRI) (Seidell, Bakker, & Kooy, 1990), there is at present no practical way to measure this depot of fat, although useful associations between body mass index and circumferences have been suggested (Kvist, Chowchuny, Grangard, Tylen, & Sjostrom, 1988). In the work of Enzi et al. (1986), lower correlations were found between subcutaneous fat at the abdominal level with abdominal visceral fat areas than for subcutaneous fat between thoracic and subcutaneous fat in the abdominal areas; the authors conclude that there is considerable independence in the relation of subcutaneous fat and visceral fat mass with increasing fatness. In addition, Després et al. (1990) show substantial adverse differences in lipoprotein profiles of a sample of obese women with almost twice the abdominal fat as another obese sample with less abdominal fat. They emphasized the need to verify these observations on men and indicate that the association between fatness and visceral fat depots is greater in men than in women, implying that obese men may not vary in their fat distribution to the extent of women. Based on a review of the literature, Desprès et al. (1990) propose a working classification of obesity to reflect different degrees of risk for cardiovascular diseases (see Table 5.2). At highest risk of disease are individuals with high levels of both subcutaneous and visceral trunk fat.

   Després et al. (1990) review several limitations of research using waist-to-hip ratio as the only measure of fat distribution, and they recommend that future research should include trunk and abdominal skinfolds and total body fat along with waist and hip circumferences. Computer tomography or magnetic resonance imaging must be included, to obtain visceral fat. Short of this but in line with the Després et al. (1990) is the research Terry, Wood, Haskell, Stefanick, and

Table 5.2 Working Classification of Fat Distribution, Obesity, and Cardiovascular Risk

Gluteal-femoral obesity	Risk of CVD	Trunk-abdominal obesity	Risk of CVD
High levels of subcutaneous fat in the hip and buttock region without excessive trunk abdominal fat	+	High levels of subcutaneous fat without accumulation of visceral fat	++
		High levels of deep abdominal fat without excessive subcutaneous fat	+++
		High levels of both subcutaneous fat and visceral fat	++++

Note. Adapted from Després et al. (1990).

Krauss (1989), where waist-to-hip ratio, subscapular-to-tricep skinfold ratio, percent body fat, and body mass index are correlated with blood lipid and lipoprotein subfractions in adult men. The authors conclude that there may be a different relationship between central obesity (as measured by the ratio of subscapular to triceps skinfold thickness) and intra-abdominal obesity (as measured by the ratio of waist to hip circumference) with lipoprotein profiles, with both ratios correlating more closely than overall body fatness to blood lipid and lipoprotein factions. Because the lipolytic activity of adipocytes at peripheral locations may differ from abdominal visceral adipocyte activity, they speculate that the correlation between abdominal and subscapular skinfolds with plasma triglycerides and VLDL and not with triceps and thigh skinfolds may be due, in part, to locational differences (peripheral vs. central) in lipolytic activity.

Future Research Directions With Fat Distribution

There are three levels of investigation, which shows the need for additional measures of fat distribution in future studies. The Level 1 method uses large samples of trunk and extremity skinfolds, waist and hip circumferences, total body fat, body mass index, and regional impedance. Although Level 1 methods can be more easily used in large samples, Level 2 methods (more direct measures of fat distribution) can also be used. The Level 2 method uses intermediate sample of sizes and estimates regional fat by dual energy radiograpy. Després et al. (1990) recommended that future research use proper body fatness and fat distribution variables for the assessment of various obesity components. However, without use of CT or MRI, the assessment of visceral abdominal fat cannot be directly made, and because CT involves considerable radiation exposure, its use in research studies will be limited to relatively small samples (Level 3 investigation with more exact measures of fat distribution). The Level 3 method uses smaller samples than in Level 2, plus regional fat estimates by computerized tomography or magnetic resonance imaging. However, given two or three successful validation studies using CT, DER, and anthropometry, I predict that the regional trunk estimates of fatness in the abdominal area by dual energy radiography (DRA) will yield valid estimates of abdominal fat, and by correcting these estimates for variation in subcutaneous abdominal skinfolds, an indirect estimate of visceral abdominal fat may be forthcoming for Level 2 investigations such as those of Terry et al. (1989). In addition, if trunk impedance measures can be shown to yield reliable estimates of trunk fat or trunk FFB, such measurements may enable more accurate estimates of internal fat distribution than waist-to-hip ratio and can also be used in Level 2 investigations (see Table 5.3).

Table 5.3   Recommended Measure for Fat Distribution for Further Research Designs Using Different Sample Sizes

	Level one (large sample size)	Level two (intermediate sample size)	Level three (small sample size)
Trunked and extremity skinfolds	✓	✓	✓
Waist and hip circumference	✓	✓	✓
Total body fat	✓	✓	✓
Body mass index	✓	✓	✓
Regional impedance	✓	✓	✓
Regional fat by dual energy radiography (DRA)		✓	✓
Regional fat by computerized tomography			✓

Summary

The various ways of assessing fat distribution are reviewed, and the conceptual systems for classifying obesity, including central versus peripheral, upper versus lower trunk adiposity, and visceral abdominal versus gluteal-femoral, are examined. The limitations in the waist-to-hip ratio are now evident, not in terms of predicting risk factors of various chronic diseases, but in the fact that this ratio includes different types of fat depots that are confounded with overall body fatness and with body size, so that from a scientific standpoint it is difficult to determine which fat depot is contributing to the underlying risk. Emerging from recent investigations into the association of coronary heart disease and fat distribution is the need to study central versus peripheral obesity as well as upper and lower trunk obesity and to use several indices of fat distribution in the same sample, as illustrated by the research of Terry et al. (1989). The validation of trunk impedance and regional dual energy radiography may enable more direct estimates of abdominal fat and allow for quantitative separation of subcutaneous and visceral abdominal fat with minimal radiation exposure. Such a development in methodology could lead to a clarification of the association of fat distribution versus total body fatness in relation to the risk of disease with the different types of obesity and fat distribution. Further analysis clarifying the extent of individual differences in fat distribution, independent of body fatness,and their association with cardiovascular risk factors is essential once better methods are developed for assessing fat distribution. In terms of risk for disease, it would appear a higher priority at this time to establish the extent of variation in the visceral abdominal fat, and its malleability with intervention in the adult male and female populations, than to resolve the central versus peripheral subcutaneous fat distribution controversy.

Chapter 6

Estimating Body Composition in Children and the Elderly

Prepubescent children have been shown to be chemically immature; as a result, adult body composition equations overestimate the fat content of children and prevalence of obesity during childhood. In recent years new body composition equations for children have been developed and are becoming widely used. In the elderly the impact of changes in chemical fat-free body composition for the two component model is controversial and not yet well established.

In my own career in assessing body composition in children and the elderly, I was involved, from 1969 to 1984, in the summer youth fitness research program at the University of Illinois, Urbana-Champaign, which was sponsored by the Physical Fitness Research Laboratory of the Department of Physical Education. Each summer 100 to 150 children between 6 and 14 years of age took part in an activity program 4 hours per day for 4 days a week. As a part of the program, selected children came to the Physical Fitness Research Laboratory, where they took part in various research studies. Many children returned to the fitness program each year, so that in time we developed a longitudinal as well as a cross-sectional data base. My four children went through the program, each attending 3 to 5 years, and I observed their changes in body composition and their development over the years. In recent years I have investigated the body composition of the elderly with my colleague Scott Going at the University of Arizona. Though much of this chapter is devoted to the problem of assessing body composition in children, the same problems are briefly examined for the elderly.

A decade earlier, my colleague Charles Tipton worked closely with D.M. Hall at the College of Agriculture at the University of Illinois. Each summer as a part of the 4-H program, they measured thousands of children to estimate their optimal weight using various skeletal dimensions. These experiences at Illinois helped shape our careers, which crossed in the 1980s and led to the development of valid equations for estimating minimal weight in the high school wrestlers population (chapter 10). In this chapter I review the development of body composition assessment in children and some of the critical studies leading to a more valid body composition equation.

Developing Body Composition Skinfold Equations for Children

In my research with the Physical Fitness Laboratory, we started with 10 skinfolds based on the research of Allen et al. (1956) and compared them with two laboratory research methods—first with body potassium (whole-body ^{40}K; Lohman, Boileau, & Massey, 1975) and later with densitometry (Boileau, Wilmore, Lohman, Slaughter, & Riner, 1981). From these large data sets we developed multiple regression equations to predict body fatness and fat-free body mass and used these equations to predict body composition in children. Most of our research was on prepubescent and pubescent children, and I supervised and measured hundreds of children for skinfolds and ^{40}K content to measure the natural-occurring radioactivity found in a relatively constant amount of all lean tissue (Lohman et al., 1975) using a whole-body liquid scintillation counter.

Using ^{40}K content to estimate fat-free body mass and percent fat, we found that the triceps and subscapular skinfolds were good sites for the estimation of fat content in 162 male children. When the ^{40}K method is used to estimate body composition, an 8-year-old male with a triceps skinfold of 7 mm, a subscapular skinfold of 6 mm, and a body weight of 28 kg would be estimated to be 17.2% fat, using this equation (Lohman et al., 1975):

$$\text{FFB, kg} = 0.87 \; wt, \text{kg} - 0.36 \; \textit{Triceps skinfold} - 0.40 \; \textit{Subscapular skinfold} + 3.7$$

$$\text{SEE} = 1.8 \text{ kg}$$

$$\% \text{ Fat} = \frac{wt - ffb}{wt} \times 100.$$

For females, we found the following equation to be predictive of FFB:

$$\text{FFB, kg} = 0.65 \; wt, \text{kg} - 0.17 \; \textit{Triceps} - 0.19 \; \textit{Subscapular} + 6.8$$

$$\text{SEE} = 2.0 \text{ kg}.$$

A female weighing 28 kg with a 10-mm tricep and 6-mm subscapular would be 20.9% fat. Using skinfolds for the 50th, 85th, and 95th percentiles (NHES, 1973), percent fat for 8 year-old male and female children was estimated (Table 6.1).

Fat-free body mass (kg) was estimated from body potassium (from whole-body ^{40}K assay), assuming boys and girls had an adult K content for fat-free mass of 2.66 g/kg, or 68.1 meq K/kg. These equations were cross-validated on another sample of boys and girls in further work by our laboratory. In time, we started

Table 6.1   Comparison of Skinfolds-Body Fat Equations With Two Criterion Methods and Adult Constants Applied to 8-Year-Old Children

Sex	Method	Percent fat at different percentiles for skinfolds[a]		
		50th	85th	95th
Males	40-K method	17.2	23.8	32.0
	Densitometry	15.4	21.1	27.3
Females	40-K method	20.9	27.7	34.0
	Densitometry	18.4	25.5	30.4

[a]Using skinfolds from the NHES (1963-1965) national probability sample and the equations for 40-K (Lohman et al., 1975) and densitometry (Boileau et al., 1981); percent fat is calculated.

to question the use of the constant 2.66 for children and presented evidence in the literature that the K content might be as low as 2.3 g/kg in children to as high as 2.7 g/kg (Slaughter, Lohman, & Boileau, 1978). If the former constant is closer to the actual value, then we would be overestimating the fat content in our sample and underpredicting FFB, kg.

In time my colleague Dick Boileau at the University of Illinois developed an underwater weighing system (designed after Akers & Buskirk, 1969), and for several years we collected ^{40}K data and body density data. We developed skinfold equations based on this approach as well, assuming the density of the fat-free body to be 1.10 g/cc, and used the Siri formula (% Fat $= \frac{4.95}{D_b} - 4.50$) to estimate body composition from body density. The following skinfold-density equation was found for 97 males (8- to 11-year-olds):

$$D_b = 1.081 - 0.0022 \ (Triceps) - 0.0019 \ (Subscapular).$$

We compared our results with another set of data by Wilmore and McNamara (1974) and found similar regression coefficients for triceps and subscapular skinfolds. Combining the two samples and using the sum of two skinfolds (linear and quadratic polynomials), we obtained the following equation:

$$\text{Density} = 1.101 - 0.0034 \ (\Sigma \ 2sk) + 0.000049 \ (\Sigma \ 2sk)^2.$$

These curvilinear lines (Boileau et al., 1981) were slightly different between samples but have been combined to yield an average equation for the purposes of illustration. Applying this equation to the same skinfolds on 8-year-old males and females yields percent fat values only slightly smaller than that found for the ^{40}K method (Table 6.1). The skinfold equation of Parízoková (1961), published several years earlier on Czechoslovakian boys, also yielded similar estimates of percent fat. Finally, the work of Forbes and Amirhakimi (1970) using skinfolds and 40-K was also found to be in agreement with our equations.

During this time period Jack Wilmore published an article on the cardiovascular risk factors in children (8 to 12 years), including blood lipids and body fatness, based on densitometry (Wilmore & McNamara, 1974). They found that the mean fat content was 18.7%, that 38% of the sample had a fat content greater than 20%, and that 13.2% of the sample had a fat content above 25%. They pointed out that the density of the fat-free body was assumed to be similar in this sample to that of young adults and that the water and bone mineral fat-free body content was similar to that of adults. They observed that "the average relative fat for college men is approximately 15%, yet they have a fatter outward appearance than these younger boys" (p. 530), adding that "additional work is needed to develop equations which will take into account these basic development differences" (Wilmore & McNamara, 1974, p. 530).

Chemical Maturity in Children

The question of chemical maturity in children needed to be tested because we realized that children may have more water and less mineral and potassium in their fat-free body than adults. The Siri formula, we suggested, would lead to an overestimation of body fatness in children, and the prevalence of obesity would be overestimated as well (Lohman, Boileau, & Slaughter, 1985). Moreover, all the work in children with ^{40}K using the constant 2.66 g/kg K content of the fat-free body may have overestimated body fatness, if the potassium content of the fat-free body increases from childhood to youth (Lohman et al., 1985).

The Foman and Haschke Line of Investigation

Earlier in this chapter we suggested that the potassium content of the fat-free body in children might vary from 2.3 g/kg FFB to 2.7 g/kg FFB, depending on which method was used to estimate fat-free body (Slaughter et al., 1978). However, it was not until research investigations were undertaken by two independent teams in the 1980s that the extent of chemical immaturity in children was established. Each group of investigators approached the question somewhat differently and, with different methods and assumptions, worked out the changes in both water and bone mineral content of the fat-free body during childhood and youth. The work of Haschke, Foman, and Ziegler (1981), Foman, Haschke, Ziegler, and Nelson (1982), and Haschke (1983a, 1983b) proceeded first to define the 9-year-old reference boy and the composition of the fat-free body (Haschke et al., 1981) from data in the literature. Soon to follow was the estimation of the body composition of reference children from birth to age 10 years (Foman et al., 1982). This work was based on data from the literature on total body water by isotope dilution, total body potassium from older-body ^{40}K assessment, total body calcium using neutron activation analysis and body density from underwater weighing using different samples of subjects. Their methods and assumptions are well documented. The body composition of adolescent males was investigated more directly by Haschke (1983a, 1983b), where body water was estimated from saliva samples using deuterium dilution in a sample of 108 boys 10 to 15 years of age. Mineral content and protein content were estimated from prediction equations of others, using height and weight. Haschke (1983b) found that water content of the fat-free body decreased from 75.2% in 10-year-old males to 73.6% in 18-year-old males, indicating that chemical maturity was not established in males until late adolescence.

The Lohman, Slaughter, and Boileau Line of Investigation

In our work with children at the University of Illinois, Dick Boileau and Mary Slaughter and I designed a study to investigate the concept of chemical maturity of children. We started with children age 7 and investigated the concept all the way into young adulthood (18- to 29-year-olds). We questioned the concept that children by the age of 5 years were chemically mature and had adult water and mineral contents of the fat-free body as Moulton (1923) had claimed for humans, largely based on animal data. We reasoned in our review article (Lohman et al., 1985) that, because of the long childhood growth phase preceding puberty, humans were not chemically mature by 4% of their life span as was the case for nonprimate mammals (Moulton, 1923).

We observed that Moulton had human data on only fetuses, infants, and young adults, and thus there was the need to investigate children and youth, especially before and after puberty. We hypothesized change not only in the water and mineral contents from prepubescence to postpubescence, but also in the potassium content of the fat-free body (Lohman et al., 1985). We set up procedures to estimate total body water from deuterium dilution using infrared spectrophotometry (Boileau et al., 1984) and bone mineral using single-beam photon absorptiometric techniques (SPA; Lohman, Slaughter, et al., 1984). For estimating the mineral content we measured the radius and ulna at the one-third distal site used by Mazess and Cameron (1971) in children and adults for estimating bone mineral content. Mazess and Cameron (1971) studied 322 children from 6 to 14 years of age and found bone mineral content to be somewhat independent of skeletal maturation.

We obtained data on children in Illinois and in Arizona from 1980 to 1983. Both black and white children were selected, and densitometry and anthropometry (Slaughter et al., 1984) were collected as well. A physical exam was also conducted, and children were classified as prepubescent, pubescent, and postpubescent based on secondary sexual characteristics (Slaughter et al., 1984).

The Bone Mineral Solution

The major challenge to the analysis of data was in the bone mineral measurement, which represented the mineral content (g/cm) of a cross-section of the radius and ulna and not the total mineral content of the body. We observed a large increase in the growth of the radius and ulna bone mineral content (g/cm) from childhood to adult in both males and females. Bone density (g/cm³) cannot be estimated using photon absorptiometry, as only the cross-sectional mineral content of a 1-cm slice of bone (g/cm) and the bone mineral content divided by width (g/cm²) of radius and ulna bone width are obtained. (For the sake of clarity, I will use *BMC* for g/cm, *BMW* for g/cm², and *BMD* for g/cm³). Part of this growth in mineral content was due to bone size and reflects larger bones, but not a relative increase in mineral content of the fat-free body, and part was due to a greater proportion of bone mineral in the fat-free body mass. Finally, a greater mineralization of bones during growth and development, leading to greater bone mineral density, was also likely to be present.

To assess the effect of bone mineral content on body density, we used multiple regression analysis in the entire sample of children and young adults. We found that association of the sum of skinfolds with body density changed with maturation, with a given skinfold corresponding to higher body density as children advanced from prepubertal to pubertal to postpubertal stages (Slaughter et al., 1984). We used nine skinfolds, four skinfolds, and two skinfolds and in each case found a significant maturation effect. Then, we added into the regression model body-water-content changes as a fraction of the fat-free body (Boileau et al., 1984) and BMC (Lohman, Slaughter, et al., 1984). We found in both the Illinois and the Arizona samples a significant effect of BMC on body density, holding skinfolds and body water content constant. The combined analysis (for Illinois and Arizona samples) was published in 1984, and a method was developed to estimate how much a change in BMC was associated with changes in density of the fat-free body (Lohman, Slaughter, et al., 1984). From this multiple regression model, we estimated the mineral content of the fat-free body in prepubescent children to be 5.2%, instead of 6.8% as in adult reference man (Brozek, et al., 1963).

In our work with body water in the same sample of children, we found water content to be 2.8% higher in prepubescent children than in young adults (Boileau et al., 1984). Thus, we proposed a water content of 76.6% and a mineral content of 5.2%, yielding a density of the fat-free body of 1.084 g/cc in prepubescent children, as compared to 73.8% water content and 6.8% mineral fat-free body content in reference man (Brozek et al., 1963). Research on body water content and its change with growth and development is presented in the following section.

Hydration in Children

The water content of the fat-free body has been estimated to be between 71% and 74% in the young adult population. Two key studies with body water content in children in the 1960s overlooked the density-water connection (see chapter 2). In the case of Young et al. (1968), low correlations were found between body water content and body density in females 9 to 16 years of age. No calculations were made in this sample of the water content of the fat-free body or of the variability of this characteristic with age. Heald et al. (1963) looked at the systematic variation of water content in the fat-free body by first estimating percent fat and fat-free body weight from body density alone in 12- to 18-year-old males. Based on these calculations they concluded that the hydration of the fat-free body was as high as 78% in 12-year-old males and decreased to 72% for 18-year-olds. Although their data do show a large change in hydration with age, it is not as dramatic if the density-water formula proposed by Siri (1961) is first used to estimate percent fat. Thus, we reanalyzed both sets of data (from Young et al., 1968, and Heald et al., 1963), using the density-water formula of Siri (1961), and found that body water as a percent of the fat-free body decreased 3.6% in males and 3% to 6% in females (Lohman et al., 1985). The work of Haschke (1983b) found the water content of the fat-free body in males decreasing from 75.2% to 73.6% from 10 to 18 years of age.

In our own work with children, we found the water content of the fat-free body to be 75.3% in the prepubertal sample as compared to 72.5% in the adult sample (Boileau et al., 1984). The decrease was similar in males (2.9%) and females (2.8%), and a significant gender effect was present with females having a higher water content than males throughout growth and development. We found the water content of the fat-free body in adults to be 73.5% for males and 74.2% for females. Combining our work (Lohman, 1986) with that of Foman et al. (1982) and Haschke (1983), I presented the following hydration results (Table 6.2) in males and females from 1 year to young adulthood (Lohman, 1989).

Table 6.2   Hydration of the Fat-Free Body in Children and Youth

Age, years	% Water content of fat-free body	
	Male	Female
1	79.0	78.8
1-2	78.6	78.5
3-5	77.8	78.3
5-6	77.0	78.0
7-8	76.8	77.6
9-10	76.2	77.0
11-12	75.4	76.6
13-14	74.7	75.5
15-16	74.2	75.0
17-20	73.8	74.5

Note. From "Assessment of Body Composition in Children" by T.G. Lohman, 1989, *Pediatric Exercise Science*, **1**, p. 21. Copyright 1989 by Human Kinetics Publishers. Adapted by permission.

Developing Skinfold Equations From Body Density, Total Body Water Content, and Total Bone Mineral Content

Given that body water and bone mineral contents of the fat-free body are changing, how can we correct our estimate of percent fat from body density to yield more accurate estimates of body fatness in children? The development of a multicomponent model including body density, body water, and bone mineral was the key to these new equations (Lohman, 1986). This development is explained in more detail in chapter 3. Here we present the equation, which can be used for children of any age (as well as adults of any age) if the density, water content, and mineral content of the body are known.

$$\% \text{ Fat} = \frac{2.749}{D_b} - 0.727 \; (w) + 1.146 \; (m) - 2.053$$

where w and b correspond to the fractions of water content and mineral content of the body, respectively.

For a prepubescent male child with a body density of 1.049 g/cc, a water content of 0.61 and a mineral content of 0.042 yield

$$\% \text{ Fat} = \frac{2.749}{1.049} - 0.727 \; (0.61) + 1.146 \; (0.042) - 2.053 = 17.2\%,$$

whereas using the 1.100 g/cc constant for fat-free body density yields

$$\% \text{ Fat} = \left(\frac{4.95}{1.049} - 4.50 \right) 100 = 21.9\%.$$

Guo, Roche and Houtkooper (1990) found that the two-component model underestimated the above multicomponent estimates of fat-free body mass by 1.5 kg to 2.0 kg in children 12 years and younger, and thus they applied a correction for the changing density of the fat-free body with age (Figure 6.1).

Using these results based on percent fat, we developed the following equations for using the sum of triceps and subscapular skinfolds with different intercepts (I) for maturation level and gender (Lohman, 1986).

$$\% \text{ Fat } = 1.35 \; (\Sigma \; 2sk) - 0.012 \; (\Sigma \; 2sk)^2 - \text{I}.$$

We then developed specific equations for each gender ($N = 310$ children and adults) and for triceps and subscapular versus triceps and calf skinfolds (Slaughter et al., 1988). The standard errors of estimate were 3.6% to 3.9% fat for the triceps plus subscapular sites and 3.8% fat for the triceps plus calf sites. In the cross-validation of these equations, we did not have other data bases with density, water, and bone, but we did obtain the large data bases of Mukherjee and Roche (1984), Harsha, Frericho, and Berenson (1978), and Lussier and Buskirk (1977) and found that for a given age and given skinfold values, our data had a lower mean body density, of 0.003 g/cc, than the other samples. We therefore adjusted all intercepts by 1.4% fat to bring our density values closer to those of others. The results are given in Table 6.3 with the final equations we published (Slaughter et al., 1988).

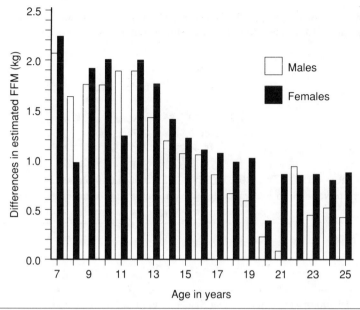

Figure 6.1   Fat-free mass. *Note*. From "Fat-Free Mass in Children and Young Adults Predicted from Biotechnic Impedance and Anthropometric Variables" by S. Guo, A.F. Roche, and L. Houtkooper, 1989, *American Journal of Clinical Nutrition*, **50**, p. 487. Copyright © 1989 by *American Journal of Clinical Nutrition*. Reprinted by permission of the American Society for Clinical Nutrition.

We discovered that for children with the sum of triceps and subscapular skinfolds above 35 mm, the curvilinear equation (X, X^2) underestimated percent fat. This was discovered when Sharon Hoerr applied our equations to an independent sample of obese adolescent females (Hoerr, Nelson, Lohman, & Steiger, 1984). After her work we realized that the curvilinear equations we developed are curvilinear in nature, and that at thick skinfolds, percent fat starts to decrease rather than increase. We found that the linear equations worked well on Dr. Hoerr's sample and that above a 35-mm skinfold the curvilinear equations start to deviate to the extent of making children with higher skinfolds have lower percent fat volumes than expected. Thus our recommendation is to use the linear equations (X only) for all children with skinfolds above 35 mm. For black children we found significantly different intercepts than for white children after adjusting for water and bone mineral content differences. For a given sum of triceps plus subscapular skinfolds, we found black males to be about 2% leaner than whites (Slaughter et al., 1988). For females, the difference was only 1%, and we have included different intercepts (2.0 vs. 3.0) to account for this difference (Table 6.3). We have developed software with all these equations, so that an individual report (see Appendix 6.1) can easily be given to each child measured for either triceps and calf or triceps and subscapular skinfolds.

Table 6.3 Prediction Equations of Percent Fat From Triceps and Calf and From Triceps and Subscapular Skinfolds in Children and Youth for Males and Females

Triceps and calf skinfolds

$$\% \text{ Fat} = 0.735 \ \Sigma SF + 1.0 \ \text{Males, all ages}$$
$$\% \text{ Fat} = 0.610 \ \Sigma SF + 5.0 \ \text{Females, all ages}$$

Triceps and subscapular skinfolds (>35 mm)

$$\% \text{ Fat} = 0.783 \ \Sigma SF + I \ \text{Males}$$
$$\% \text{ Fat} = 0.546 \ \Sigma SF + 9.7 \ \text{Females}$$

Triceps and subscapular skinfolds (<35 mm)[a]

$$\% \text{ Fat} = 1.21 \ (\Sigma SF) - 0.008 \ (\Sigma SF)^2 + I \ \text{Males}$$
$$\% \text{ Fat} = 1.33 \ (\Sigma SF) - 0.013 \ (\Sigma SF)^2 + 2.5 \ \text{Females (2.0 blacks, 3.0 whites)}$$

I = Intercept varies with maturation level and racial group for males as follows:

Age	Black	White
Prepubescent	−3.5	−1.7
Pubescent	−5.2	−3.4
Postpubescent	−6.8	−5.5
Adult	−6.8	−5.5

Note. Calculations were derived using Slaughter et al. (1988) equation.

[a]Thus for a white pubescent male with a triceps of 15 and a subscapular of 12, the % fat would be:

$$\% \text{ Fat} = 1.21 \ (27) - 0.008 \ (27)^2 - 3.4$$
$$= 23.4\%$$

Table 6.4 Estimated Density of the Fat-Free Body of Elderly Females

Young female adult (N = 55)	Age	Body weight	Fat	Water	Protein	Mineral	D_{FFB}	D_{FFB}[a]
				Percent of fat-free body				
$\overline{X}$	29.0	58.0	23.4	.721	.214	.065	1.101	1.101
S	3.9	7.0	5.2					
Elderly female adult (N = 61)								
$\overline{X}$	74.5	58.9	32.6	.712	.230	.059	1.099	1.0942
S	5.9	8.6	6.0					

Note. Calculations were derived using Heymsfield et al. (1989) equations.

[a]If the actual density of protein and mineral were to change with age as well as the fat-free body composition, then the density of the fat-free body would be lower. For example, if we assume a 5% decrease in protein and mineral density in the elderly, then I have calculated the density of the fat-free body. Whether the density of these components changes with age is unknown.

Constancy of Fat-Free Body Composition in the Elderly

In a recent review article estimating body composition in the elderly, Heymsfield, Wang, Lichtman, et al. (1989) emphasize the new advances in neutron activation analysis and dual photon absorptiometry as tools for critically evaluating the underlying assumptions for assessing body composition in the elderly. In a preliminary analysis on 61 elderly female subjects, the authors estimated the density of the fat-free body from their estimates of water, protein, and mineral, using neutron activation analysis, deuterium dilution, and dual photon absorptiometry (Table 6.4). Unlike the results with prepubescent children, the changes in fat-free body composition in this elderly sample had very little effect on the density of the fat-free body. That is because as the mineral content decreases as a fraction of the fat-free body, as in prepubescent children, the water content is also lower, in contrast to the higher water content of children. And with an increase in the protein content, the overall density of the fat-free body is only slightly lower in this elderly sample. If we assume a decrease of 5% in the density of the mineral and protein, then we would lower the density of the fat-free body to 1.0942.

$$\frac{1}{D_{FFB}} = \frac{0.712}{0.99371} + \frac{0.230}{1.27} + \frac{0.059}{2.88} = 1.0942$$

$$\frac{1}{D_{FFB}} = \frac{0.712}{0.9937} + \frac{0.230}{1.34} = \frac{0.059}{3.032} = 1.102.$$

From these results, we can see that accurately estimating the changes in the water content of the FFB is a critical factor of body composition assessment in the elderly. In a recent review of this area, Schoeller (1989) concludes that there is little change in the relationship between total body water content and fat-free mass with aging. In animal data a slight increase in water is indicated in some samples, and a decrease, in others. Thus, at present it does not appear that the chemical content of the fat-free body influences fat-free body density in the elderly to the extent it does in prepubescent children. In another review of body composition assessment in the elderly, Chumlea and Baumgartner (1989) advocate a four-component model (fat, water, protein, mineral) to establish reference data in the elderly to resolve the uncertainty in using the two-component model. With a valid body composition approach for the elderly, they advocate collecting data on large representative samples of black, white, Hispanic, and Oriental elderly to establish reference data for anthropometry and body composition.

Summary

In this chapter I have reviewed the recent developments for estimating body composition in children. Through use of the multicomponent approach to assessing body composition, it has been established that the density of the fat-free body is less than 1.100 g/cc, as in adults, and that anthropometric equations based on body density lead to overestimation of fat content in children. The development of skinfold equations in children is reviewed, and recent equations now available for children are presented. The need for further research in the elderly to determine the density of the fat-free body is critical to obtain valid estimates of body composition. Use of skinfold equations developed in the middle-aged population and elderly, assuming a constant fat-free-body density, may lead to an overestimation of body fatness due to the bone mineral loss with age; however, a decrease in the water content of the fat-free body with age lessens the bone mineral effect. Anthropometric equations using multicomponent models as a criterion method in older populations are likely to be properly developed in the near future.

APPENDIX 6.1

Sample report on fatness estimate for each child.

Body composition   An estimate

Name: Tim

Age: 12 years old   Height 60.0 in.   Weight 123.0 lbs.

Skinfolds: Tricep 34.0 mm   Calf 23.0 mm

From tricep and calf sites your percent fat can be predicted within plus or minus 3.0%.

Your percent fat from sum of triceps and calf skinfolds: 43.2%

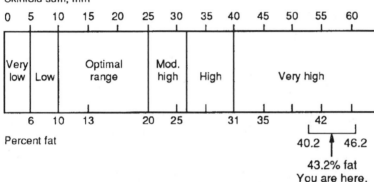

An optimal amount of fat is from 10.0% to 20.0% for boys. If you are in the optimal range, this level of fatness will support good health. If you are above the optimal range, then it would be a good idea to slowly lose excess fat by increasing your physical activity. Also eating less high-calorie foods, such as potato chips, french fries, ice cream, whole milk, butter, cream, and high fat meats will help.

Your sum of skinfolds compared with national norms on children and youth.

Percentile norms

Your sum	Norm avg.	0	10	20	30	40	50	60	70	80	90	99
57.0	22.0											

Your sum of skinfolds is less than   1% of all people.

Optimal weight range calculations:

Minimum weight	Optimal range	Maximum weight
74.4 lbs	between 77.7 and 87.4 lbs	93.2 lbs

Note. Adapted from *Body Composition Estimation for Children* [computer software] by T.G. Lohman, 1987, Champaign, IL: Human Kinetics. Copyright 1987 by Human Kinetics.

Chapter 7

The Prevalence of Obesity in Children in the United States

The prevalence of obesity throughout childhood has not been well defined because of the variety of methods and procedures used to estimate body fatness. The three major approaches—body mass index, skinfold percentiles (usually the 85th and 95th), and a cutoff value for percent body fatness—yield widely different estimates. Further, prevalence varies with region of country, ethnic group, season of year, and age of child. Finally, decade is an important factor, with recent evidence accumulating that more children in the 1980s are obese than were obese in the 1960s.

Obesity is an excess of body fat frequently resulting in a significant impairment of health. Because body fat content is not readily estimated in the field, the level of fatness at which one is at greater risk for health impairment has not been clearly established by epidemiological research, although there is overwhelming evidence that obesity has adverse effects on health and longevity. What epidemiological research does show is a relationship between body mass index (BMI) and mortality as well as risk of acquiring specific diseases (hypertension, hypercholesterolemia, cardiovascular disease, non-insulin-dependent diabetes, excessive risk of certain cancers, and other medical problems). In both males and females, increased mortality is found at a body mass index of 27, which corresponds to a body weight about 20% above desirable (Metropolitan Life Insurance Company, 1983). The National Center for Health Statistics (NCHS) has defined obesity in terms of BMI as 27.8 for men and 27.3 for women. If we can convert BMI to percent body fatness, then we can begin to establish a percent-fat standard for defining risk for disease and greater mortality. Ideally, however, we need epidemiological studies using more direct methods of estimating percent fat than BMI, because of its insensitivity to obesity and the confounding factors associated with lean body size, frame size, and leg length, as discussed in chapter 4.

Developing Fat Standards in Adults

Using BMIs of 27.8 for men and 27.3 for women, we can estimate a corresponding fat content of 25 ± 2% for men and 32 ± 2% for women, based on several research studies cited in chapter 4. We also know that a young adult man averages about 15% fat, based on body density, and young adult women, about 25%. Because women may have a lower bone mineral content than men, the Siri formula overestimates percent fat for females by about 2%. Thus, the mean fat content for women is likely to be closer to 23% (Figure 7.1); however, gender differences in bone mineral content of fat-free body are not well established (chapter 3).

Given these standards for percent fat, we can describe the prevalence of obesity in children and youth if we use 25% fat for males and 32% for females. With this definition in mind, I published (Lohman et al., 1989) the results, using the triceps and subscapular skinfolds, on the NHANES I (1971-1975; Johnson, Fulword, Abraham, & Brymer, 1981) survey and the Slaughter et al. equations (1988), which were developed specifically for children and youth (chapter 6). For these data we can see that the prevalence of obesity is fairly low in early childhood (5% or less), increases in youth and young adulthood, and reaches greatest prevalence in middle-aged adults (Lohman, 1989). Colleagues and I described the basis for this approach in a research paper (Lohman, Going, Slaughter, & Boileau, 1989) using the NCHS data of 1971-1974 (Johnson, Fulword, Abraham, & Brymer, 1981). We found that 6- to 8-year-old males were only 17.2% and 23.3% fat at the 85th and 95th skinfold percentiles, respectively, and that the prevalence of males above 25% fat was much lower than usually estimated.

This approach to the definition of obesity in terms of percent fat, 25% for males and 32% fat for females, is new and has not yet been widely used, because of the long tradition of using body weight and height or, more recently, skinfold percentiles. However, as more accurate body composition methods are developed and adopted by various professionals, it is likely that this approach using percent fat will be widely used in the coming years by physicians, pediatricians, physical educators, nutritionists, exercise physiologists, and human biologists. The concept

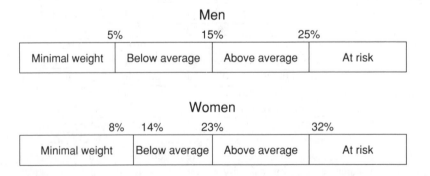

Figure 7.1   Percent body fat standards for men and women in relation to health.

is sound; only the actual levels need further research, so that different levels of body fatness can be identified with different risks of disease, and fat distribution can be separated from total body fatness and assessed as an independent risk factor (see chapter 5). Thus, the risk of maintaining 20% to 25% fat, 25% to 30% fat, 30% to 35% fat, versus 35% to 40% fat needs to be assessed in males and females for a better definition of excess body fatness and its relation to health. For example, future research using measures of body fatness such as skinfolds or bioelectric impedance may show that males between 20% and 25% fat have greater risks of mortality, or more cardiovascular risk factors, than men between 10% and 15% or between 15% and 20%. Thus the Figure 7.1 modification to encourage men to decrease body fat content to 20% rather than 25%.

Skinfold Percentiles as a Standard for Assessing Obesity

Alternative to the use of percent fat as a standard for obesity, skinfold percentiles have been used because of the difficulty of estimating body composition in children (see chapter 6). Triceps skinfolds and both the 85th and 95th percentile have been used by Dietz and Gortmaker (1984) and Gortmaker, Dietz, Sobol, & Wheler (1987), who have shown that the prevalence of obesity has increased from 1963 to 1980 and that it is affected by regions of the country, season, population density, and racial background. In 6- to 11-year-olds, the prevalence varied from 23% in the Northeast to 14% in the West, from 23% in metropolitan areas to 16% in rural areas, by season (highest in winter, lowest in summer), and by racial background (higher in whites than in nonwhites).

Using the 85th percentile for triceps skinfold, Gortmaker et al. (1987) showed that more children between 6 and 11 years, as well as between 12 and 17 years, were above the 85th percentile in 1971-1974 and 1976-1980 as compared to 1963-1965. For the 6- to 11-year-olds, Gortmaker et al. (1987) found a 61% increase for boys and a 46% increase in girls. That is, whereas 17.9% of the male sample had a triceps skinfold greater than the 85th percentile in 1963-1965, by 1976-1980, 28.9% of the same age and sex were above the triceps skinfold value, for a 61% increase (Table 7.1). Thus, the prevalence of obesity, using triceps skinfold, changed from about 1 in 6 to slightly more than 1 in 4 for this age group of males. For older children (12 to 17 years), Gortmaker found that the boys increased only 18% compared to a 58% increase in girls. Gortmaker et al. (1987) also found a lower prevalence of obesity in blacks than in whites; however, the rate of increase in prevalence was greater for blacks over the 15-year period. In addition to the 85th percentile of the criterion for obesity, Gortmaker also used the 95th percentile and found even greater percentage increases in children exceeding the 95th percentile over the 15-year period.

It is important to establish how fat children are at a given age (percent body fatness) when they exceed the 85th and 95th percentiles for skinfolds, to interpret the findings of Gortmaker et al. (1987). To this end I developed Table 7.2 to show how much body-fat content varies at the 50th, 85th, and 95th percentiles for age and gender in the NHANES 1963-1965 sample. I based this table on the triceps and subscapular norms that I developed from the data base (NHES, 1973), much the same way as Gortmaker had done with triceps alone. Then I converted the sum of the two skinfolds to percent fat using the equations of Slaughter et al. (1988). Figure 7.2 shows results for the 85th percentile.

Table 7.1   Increase in the Prevalence of Obesity (Gortmaker et al., 1987)

Age group	1963-1965	1976-1980	% Increase
6- to 11-year-olds			
Boys	17.9%	28.9%	61%
Girls	17.3%	25.2%	46%
12- to 17-year-olds			
Boys	15.5%	18.3%	18%
Girls	16.1%	25.5%	58%

Note. Prevalence of obesity based on triceps skinfold (NHES, 1963-1965).

Table 7.2   Percent Fat Corresponding to the 50th, 85th, and 95th Percentiles for Triceps Plus Subscapular Skinfolds

	Males				Females	
	Percentiles				Percentiles	
50th		85th	95th	50th	85th	95th
Age, years Σ2SK	% Fat	Σ2SK	% Fat	Σ2SK	% Fat	Σ2SK	% Fat	Σ2SK	% Fat	Σ2SK	% Fat

Age, years	Σ2SK	% Fat	Σ2SK	% Fat	Σ2SK	% Fat	Σ2SK	% Fat	Σ2SK	% Fat	Σ2SK	% Fat
6	12	11.7	16	15.6	20	19.6	14	13.5	19	18.1	27	23.9
8	13	12.7	19	18.4	28	25.9	16	15.5	25	22.6	36	29.4
10	14	12.7	24	21.9	33	28.8	18	17.2	31.6	26.5	43	33.2
12	14.5	12.5	27	23.6	44	35.0	19.5	18.5	34	27.7	47.3	35.5
14	14	11.0	26.5	22.0	39	30.5	23.5	21.6	37.5	30.2	52.6	38.4
16	14	9.0	24	18.9	39	29.3	25.5	23.0	42	32.6	58	41.4

Males: For 6- and 8-year-olds, the intercept was −1.7, for 10-year-olds, −2.5; for 12-year-olds, −3.4; for 14-year-olds, −4.4; and for 16-year-olds, −5.5; and the equation is % fat = 1.21 Σ2SK − 0.008 (Σ2SK) 2 + I. For males with skinfolds greater than 35 mm, % fat = 0.783 (Σ2SK) + 2.2 (6- to 8-year-olds), 0.6 (10- to 12-year-olds), and −1.2 (14- to 16-year-olds).

Females: % Fat = 1.33 (Σ2SK) − 0.013 (Σ2SK) 2 − 2.5 (one intercept for all ages). For females with skinfolds greater than 35 mm, % fat = 0.546 (Σ25K) + 9.7, all ages.

Note. Calculations were derived using NHES norms (1963-1965), computed from data obtained from the NHES (1973).

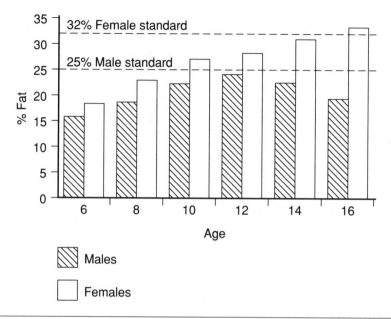

Figure 7.2   Percent fat for children of different ages at the 85th percentile of triceps plus subscapular skinfolds. *Note.* Data from NHES (1973).

We can observe from Table 7.2 that boys at the 85th percentile for triceps plus subscapular are 15.6% fat at 6 years of age to 23.6% at 12 years of age. For girls the 85th percentile for triceps plus subscapular is equivalent to 18.1% fat and continues to rise to 32.6% for 16-year-olds (Table 7.2, Figure 7.2). Thus, the same skinfold percentile at a given age varies considerably in fat content, and for skinfold percentiles to be used in establishing the prevalence of obesity, we must define obesity as varying from 15.6% fat in 6-year-old males to 32.6% fat for 16-year-old females. Such a variation in standards is a limitation in skinfold percentiles and should lead us away from using them in the future to estimate the prevalence of obesity. To use one standard for all children regardless of age is a better method for defining obesity, and now that body fatness can be estimated in children of all ages with skinfold-to-body-fat equations, we propose that the charts in Figures 7.3 and 7.4 be utilized for both future research studies, to define risks at each level of fatness, and for clinical evaluation of individual children. These charts were derived from the equations presented in chapter 6 and published by Slaughter et al. (1988). The equations are more exact than the charts, because of the small change in the relation of skinfolds to percent fat by age as shown in chapter 6. The development and use of these charts is further explained in Lohman (1987). Software developed by myself and my son, Mike Lohman, is available from Human Kinetics for the microcomputer (IBM or Apple). Appendix 6.1 shows sample output for this software package.

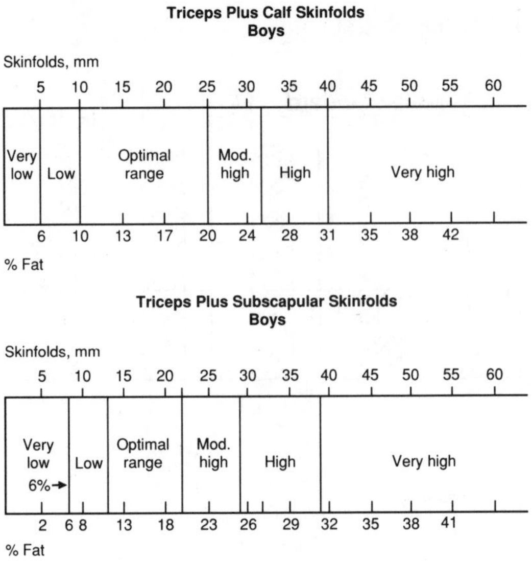

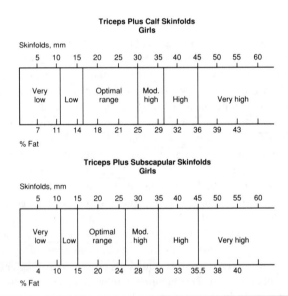

Figure 7.3 Percent-fat charts for boys. *Note.* From *Measuring Body Fat Using Skinfolds* [videotape] by T.G. Lohman, 1987, Champaign, IL: Human Kinetics. Copyright 1987 by a Human Kinetics. Printed by permission.

Figure 7.4 Percent-fat charts for girls. *Note.* From *Measuring Body Fat Using Skinfolds* [videotape] by T.G. Lohman, 1987, Champaign, IL: Human Kinetics. Copyright 1987 by Human Kinetics. Printed by permission.

New Percent-Fat Standards for Children

Research on children and youth, as well as adults, needs to be conducted to develop percent-fat standards in relation to health. In the pioneering work of Berenson, McMahon, and Voors (1980), children and youth have been studied in Bogalusa, Louisiana, for the past 20 years, relating skinfolds to cardiovascular risks factors including blood pressure levels (Aristimuno, Foster, Voors, Srinivasan, & Berenson, 1984; Smoak, Burke, Freedman, Webber, & Berenson, 1987), blood lipids (Aristimuno et al., 1984; Berenson et al., 1982), and glucose tolerance (Voors, Harsha, Rachakishmamurtz, Srinivasan, & Berenson, 1982).

The studies clearly show that skinfolds are related to an increased risk for higher levels of lipids, lipoproteins, blood pressure levels, and glucose tolerance and that, already in childhood, cardiovascular risk factors are developing with a greater probability in fatter children. Based on these findings, my colleagues Scott Going and Dan Williams and I acquired part of the data base of blood pressure and blood lipids from the Bogalusa Heart Study for the years 1983 through 1985 in cooperation with Dr. Berenson. We converted skinfolds to percent fat, using the equations developed in chapter 6, and related risk for elevation of blood pressure and serum lipids to percent fat. Our thinking was to test for differences in the prevalence of cardiovascular risk factors at different levels of body fatness. We used the uppermost quintile as an index of elevated blood pressure, total cholesterol, and serum lipoprotein ratio in a biracial sample of 1,667 males and 1,653 females between 5 and 18 years of age. Thirty-seven percent of the sample was black, the remaining were white. We found more than 20% representation in the upper quintile for boys above 25% fat, and for girls, above 30% fat, accounting for age, race, fasting status, and trunkal fat patterning (ratio of triceps to subscapular skinfolds) (Williams et al., 1992). The mean results of all five indices of risk—systolic and diastolic blood pressure, total cholesterol, and lipoprotein cholesterol ratios (LDL-C/HDI-C and VLDL-C + LDL-C/HDL-C)—show risk in the upper quintile with percent fat (Figure 7.5) above 25% fat for males and 30% for females. This is the first direct evidence linking a percent-fat level to risk of coronary heart disease in children.

Increased Obesity in Children During the 1980s

Evidence of the increase in the prevalence of obesity in the U.S. population is further confirmed by data obtained in the 1980s as part of the National Children's Youth Fitness Study (NCYFS, 1985). We have already discussed the evidence for the increase during the 1970s based on the triceps skinfold at the NHANES II (Gortmaker et al., 1987) as compared to data obtained in the 1960s (NHES national probability sample, 1973). For the NCYFS comparison (1985) with the NHES (1960s), we used triceps and subscapular skinfolds as well as body mass index to test two hypotheses: (a) The prevalence of obesity is higher in the 1980s than it was in the 1960s, and (b) Children are fatter at all percentiles in the 1980s as compared to the 1960s. Both samples involved 500 subjects per age group for

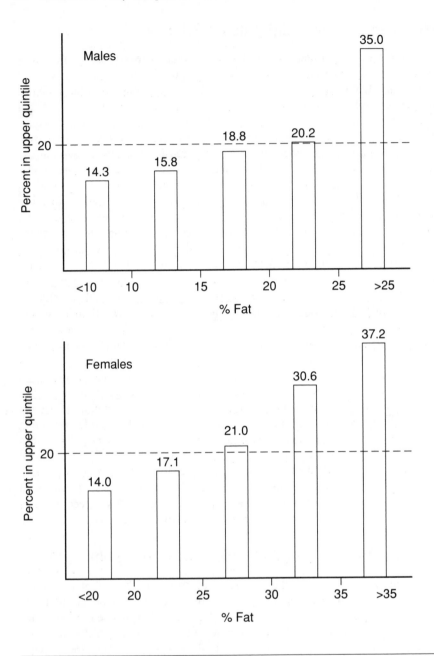

Figure 7.5   Percent of children and adolescents classified in the upper quintile based on the mean of five cardiovascular variables with percent body fat.

both boys and girls, in contrast to the smaller samples of Gortmaker et al. (1987) (NHANES II of less than 200 per age group) and thus provide an excellent sample size for the estimation in the changes in prevalence of obesity. The major findings have recently been completed (Lohman et al., 1992) and indicate that for both skinfolds, using the triceps plus subscapular percentile (85th), and for body mass index percentiles (85th), in boys and girls 6 to 11 years old the prevalence in obesity has increased 62% and 65%, respectively; and in boys and girls 6 to 11 years old, by 55% and 44%, respectively (BMI at 85th percentile). These results are similar to those of the 1970s sample (NHANES II) and compare favorably with the Gortmaker et al. (1987) estimates. Because a greater number of children exceed the 85th and 95th levels for both indices, we have confirmation that the increase in fatness is actually the case and not some artifact of a skinfold measurement procedure. Also, the fact that two different sampling methods (NCYFS vs. NHES) for establishing national probability samples in the 1970s and 1980s showed comparable results further substantiates the findings of Gortmaker et al. (1987).

If there are more children above the 85th and 95th percentiles for skinfolds in the 1980s, what about skinfolds at all percentiles? Are children fatter at all levels, or is the increase in fatness seen only at the upper end of the distribution? Figure 7.6 shows how the answers depend on age, with greater differences in the younger children and fewer differences in the older children, especially at 15 to 17 years of age. Both the 6- to 9-year-old and 10- to 12-year-old children are fatter throughout the distribution, with a further shift on the prevalence above the 85th and 95th percentiles. For the 13- to 14-year-olds and 15- to 17-year-olds, boys are fatter at all percentiles except the 95th. For 13- to 14-year-old girls, the 1980 sample is fatter at all levels except at the 85th and 95th percentiles. For these 15- to 17-year-olds we see that even at the 75th percentile the fatness-by-decade pattern changes.

Because weight and height were obtained for each child as well as skinfolds, we can compare the body mass index for each age group and at each percentile to compare our estimates of prevalence of obesity with BMI. In a detailed analysis (Lohman et al., 1992), we found similar results. Children are significantly heavier for their height at all ages except for 16- and 17-year-old girls, and the prevalence of obesity based on BMI percentile is significantly greater at all ages up to 13 years (Lohman et al., 1992). When the young children showed greater differences in skinfolds and a higher prevalence of obesity, similar results were found using BMI. Thus, we can conclude that both indices of fatness—BMI and skinfolds—show comparable results, with obesity on the increase in the 1980s for all children up to 15 years of age.

New Estimates for the Prevalence of Obesity Based on Fat Content

If we convert skinfolds to percent fat for the 6-year-old population in 1963-1965 (NHES, 1973), we find that only 2% of boys exceed 25% fat and 5% of girls

Males

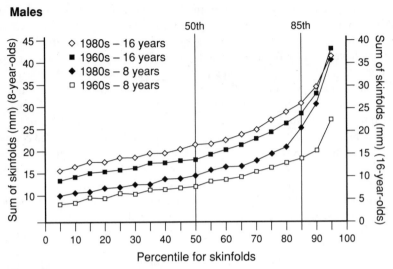

Females

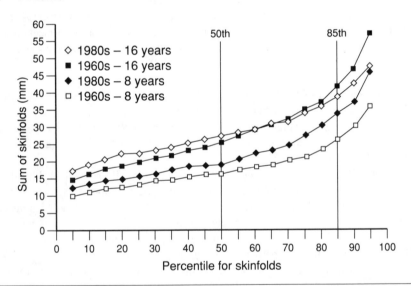

Figure 7.6   Percentile for skinfolds in (a) males and (b) females.

exceed 32% fat. For the NCYFS 1985 sample, we found that 5% of boys are above 25% fat and 9% of girls are above 32% fat (Table 7.3). Similarly we can convert skinfolds to percent fat to estimate the prevalence of obesity at other age groups based on our definitions of obesity as 25% fat for males and 32% fat for females (Table 7.3). We see that the prevalence of obesity rises rapidly from 6 to 12 years in boys and then decreases and continues to rise to 40% for 14- and

Table 7.3   Prevalence of Obesity Based on 25% Fat for Males and 32% for Females

Age, years	Males NHES	Males NCYFS	Females NHES	Females NCYFS
6	2%	6%	5%	9%
8	5%	12%	10%	20%
10	10%	16%	17%	20%
12	13%	19%	20%	25%
14	10%	12%	30%	40%
16	8%	8%	40%	40%

Note. Data from NHES (1973) and NCYHS (1985).

16-year-old girls. These results are the first estimates of obesity from the NCYFS data and show the contrast between gender during the adolescent years, with less than 10% of male adolescents being above 25% fat but 40% of female adolescents being above 32% fat.

Summary

In this chapter I have defined obesity in terms of percent fat as 25% fat for males and 32% fat for females. I have shown that skinfold percentiles correspond to a different level of fatness for a given age and are not an ideal method to study the prevalence of obesity. Based on the national norms for skinfolds and the above definition of obesity, the prevalence of obesity increases from childhood to youth and has increased from the 1960s to the 1980s. This increase is further documented by increases in BMI and skinfold percentiles in both boys and girls. A major thesis of this chapter is the need to use percent-fat standards and skinfold equations in assessing obesity in future clinical and research studies as well as in field tests of body composition assessment on children. A great challenge lies ahead if we are to reverse the trend toward a higher prevalence of childhood obesity in the coming years in the U.S. population.

Chapter 8

Tracking and Body Fatness

Strategies for intervention in and prevention of obesity depend, in part, on the degree of tracking of this trait, or the consistency with which a given level of fatness is maintained throughout childhood and adolescence into adulthood. Estimates of tracking and the hereditability of body fatness are controversial and need to be resolved in the coming decade with improved methodologies and designs, so that more effective intervention studies and strategies for the prevention of obesity can be discovered.

The degree to which body fatness tracks from infancy to adulthood is important to understand. We need to know the developmental aspects of obesity and decide at what age intervention programs should be implemented to decrease the incidence and prevalence of childhood obesity. For example, if obesity tracks strongly from infancy to childhood to adulthood, then it would be effective to delineate specific subgroups of young children who are obese and develop intervention programs specifically for this group, as illustrated by the recent 10-year follow-up of family-based treatment for obese children (Epstein, Valoski, Wing, & McCurly, 1990). If, on the other hand, obesity does not track strongly, as suggested by the 20-year follow-up study of Garn and Lavelle (1985), this means that most children who are obese at any given age do not remain so over time and that many nonobese children become obese during childhood and adolescence. If the incidence of obesity (the number of new cases of obesity occurring over a given period of time) is high throughout the developmental years, intervention programs need to be available to all children. That is, obesity can develop at any age, given the presence of certain as yet not well-defined contributors, including physical inactivity, family and cultural eating patterns, genetic predisposition and individual personality characteristics and behaviors.

Research Studies With Tracking

Research with infants, children, and adolescents has used skinfolds and body mass index to follow the extent of obesity tracking over several years. Roche (1985), reviewing the earlier literature, concluded that the relationship of obesity at birth to obesity at older ages is very low and that correlations between measures of obesity before 9 years of age and the same measure at 16 years are low.

Tracking in Infancy and Childhood

In a 20-year follow-up study by Garn and Lavelle (1985) using skinfolds, only 26% of the obese childhood sample (383 children between 0.5 and 5.5 years) were found to be obese as adults, with the expected percent by chance to be 15%. Obesity was defined as above the 85th percentile for age and sex for triceps and subscapular skinfolds. Similar results were found for each skinfold site.

In the 20-year follow-up, the correlation between skinfolds at an early age and at a 20-year interval was 0.13 for triceps and 0.16 for subscapular ($N = 383$). Thus, the initial childhood measurement accounted for less than 2% of the variation in the follow-up adult measurement, showing almost no predictive value. Of the children in the lean sample (15th percentile), only 15% remained in that category 20 years later, as expected just by chance. Thus, the tracking of a lean child is essentially zero and not associated with a higher probability of being lean as an adult. The fatness distribution of adults who were lean as children overlaps considerably with the fatness distribution of those who were obese as children.

The results of the 56 lean children in the lean sample showed that 36 increased their fatness by one to three standard deviations. The results for the initially obese group of children showed that only 7 out of 47 became fatter relative to the adult obese group, and 24 became leaner by more than one standard deviation. Still, 26% of the children designated initially obese remained obese after 20 years and, relative to the initially nonobese, were 1.77 times more likely to become obese adults. The key question for future research is "why some obese infants and children remain obese while most become less than obese by early adulthood" (Garn & Lavelle, 1985).

Kramer, Barr, Leduc, Boisjoly, and Pless (1985) looked at 347 infants measured at 6, 12, and 24 months for body weight, body mass index, and sum of three skinfolds (triceps, subscapular, and suprailiac). From this data one can see that body fatness tracks to some extent between 6 months and 2 years of age, with a correlation of 0.53 for the sum of three skinfolds. Thus, 27% of the variation in body fatness at 2 years of age can be accounted for by fatness at 6 months. In multiple regression analysis, high birth weights, shorter duration of breast feeding, sex (female), and higher maternal relative weight could account for only 10% of the variation in skinfolds at 2 years of age. Thus, in the early development of the child, much of the variation in fatness cannot be accounted for by the variables under study, and already after 2 years, fatness at 6 months and fatness at 24 months were not closely associated. In a study on body fatness and physical activity (Berkowitz, Agras, Korner, Kraemer, & Zeanah, 1985) in 52 children between 4 and 8 years of age, parental obesity and daytime physical activity could account for 30% of the variation in the child's adiposity and were more closely associated with body fatness than various measures of infant fatness and infant activity level during the first 30 days of life. The authors call attention to the need for longitudinal studies relating physical activity and fatness over the first few years of life.

Tracking in Adolescence

We have seen in infants and young children that obesity tracks only to a limited extent and that the majority of obese infants and young children become nonobese by young adulthood. Because many young children classified as obese by the 85th-percentile standard are not very fat in terms of an absolute level of fat content (the 85th percentile for a 6- to 8-year-old corresponds to a fat content of 17% for males and 22% for females; Lohman et al., 1989), part of the explanation for low tracking comes from the lack of obese children in terms of percent fat in infants and children. Thus, if only those children above 25% fat for males and 32% for females were identified, the degree of tracking in young children may be higher. What about older children and youth? Does tracking become more predominant in their age group? Evidence from the Bogalusa Heart Study is that obesity tracks to a greater extent in older children and children with a greater degree of initial obesity (95th percentile vs. 85th percentile for triceps skinfold). In a 9-year follow-up study by Freedman et al. (1987) on 1,490 black and white children of both genders and initially distributed over ages 2 to 14 years, we can see a higher association between triceps skinfolds in 11- to 14-year-olds ($r = .57$) versus 2- to 4-year-olds ($r = .45$). That is, the triceps skinfold in the 11- to 14-year-old group was more predictive of triceps skinfold in this same group 9 years later (aged 18 to 23). In this sample of 1,490 children, 222 were initially identified as obese (above the 85th percentile). Freedman et al. (1987) found that 66% of the children with a greater degree of initial obesity remained obese 8 years later (49 of 74 children with triceps greater than the 95th percentile at a given age) as compared to the 32% of children with a moderate degree of initial obesity who remained obese after 9 years (47 of 148 children with triceps between the 85th and 95th percentiles). We can estimate that prepubescent boys above the 85th percentile are above 17% fat and that those above the 95th percentile are more than 23% fat. For girls, the corresponding values are 22% and 27% (Lohman et al., 1989).

Besides age, there are other variables, such as gender and ethnic group, that might significantly affect the degree of tracking in children and youth. Freedman et al. (1987) found the highest tracking of skinfolds in black females ($r = .64$) as compared to the lowest in white females ($r = .45$). Black males tracked with an r of .59; white males, .52. Thus, cultural factors may well enter into the development of obesity, with these factors being different in the white female population than in the black female population.

Another interesting observation from the Bogalusa Heart Study is the tracking of fatness in the very lean. Of the initial 223 subjects identified as below the 15th percentile, 41% remained in that category after 8 years. In contrast with the results on lean infants who did not track at all in the 20-year follow-up study of Garn and Lavelle (1985), the predictive values of the 85th and the 15th percentiles are about the same, suggesting that changes in body composition in both groups classified as obese and lean are the rule rather than the exception.

Twin Studies and Body Fatness

Two recent studies on the genetic aspects of obesity appear to support the concept of tracking from a genetic standpoint. In the first study, by Stunkard, Jennifer, Harris, Pedersen, and McClearn (1990), 93 pairs of identical twins who were reared apart were compared to 154 pairs of identical twins reared together. Body mass index was used as the estimate of body composition. The intrapair correlation of 93 pairs was .70 for males and .66 for females and similar to the 154 pairs of twins reared together ($r = .74$, males; $r = .77$, females). Much lower correlations were found for samples of dizygotic twins raised together and apart (r ranged from .15 to .33). The authors conclude that sharing the same childhood environment did not contribute to the similarity of body mass index of twins later in life and that genetic factors appear to be major determinants of body mass index, with as much as 70% of the variance accounted for in Western society. The results, however, apply to body mass index over the normal range in the population with few obese twins represented in the sample. In a second study, by Bouchard et al. (1990), 12 pairs of young adult male monozygotic twins were overfed 1,000 kcal/day for 100 days. Body weight increased from as little as 4.3 kg in one twin pair to as much as 13.3 kg in another twin pair. The authors found evidence for genetic factors, especially the genetics-by-environment interaction, to explain the 3 times more variance among pairs in body composition changes than within pairs, with certain genotypes responding to an excessive caloric intake with a large weight gain and other genotypes responding with limited weight gain. Because subjects averaged 11% fat at the beginning of the study and 18% fat after 100 days of overfeeding, conclusions can be extended only to a nonobese population.

Cultural and Environmental Factors

Two studies on the influence of a common environment and the development of obesity offer contrasting views. Stunkard et al. (1986) concluded from a sample of 540 adult Danish adoptees representing four weight classes, based on body mass index, that genetic influences have an important role in determining human fatness in adults and that family environment alone has no apparent effect. They found no relation between weight class of the adoptee and the body mass index of her or his adoptive parent, whereas the relationship between the weight class of adoptee and body mass index of his or her biological parent was associated with obese adoptees having biological parents with significantly higher BMI than nonobese adoptees. Although Stunkard et al. (1986) emphasized that lack of environmental effect in the population under study, they are careful to point out that the findings do not mean that body fatness is not influenced by environment. This population of Denmark twins represents a Western society with an abundance of food, and their findings may be dependent on a genetics-environment interaction. They point out that a different level of genetic influence might result in different circumstances; thus, "we do not know how a genetic predisposition to fatness may be affected by environmental factors" (p. 196). They go on to state that if family environment alone has no role in obesity, efforts should be directed toward persons with greater risk of obesity rather than toward all children. Quoting Mayer (1965), "Eighty percent of the offspring of two obese parents become obese as compared to 14 percent of the offspring of two parents of normal weight" (p. 413). Thus, to decrease adult obesity, Stunkard recommended, we should identify children at risk based on parental obesity and target this subpopulation for prevention of this disorder. A 10-year follow-up of such an attempt (Epstein et al., 1990) shows that obese children from families with one or more obese parents were less obese after 10 years when assigned to a family-based treatment program for both parents and children, than obese children without such an intervention program for their parents. The treatment program consisted of diet, exercise, and behavior management training with reinforcement for weight loss and behavior change, using eight weekly treatment meetings and six additional meetings distributed over 6 months. This unique study with a 10-year follow-up provides the first evidence that treatment of childhood obesity can produce effects that persist into young adulthood. Stunkard and Berkowitz (1990) acknowledge, "The increase in childhood obesity cries out for intervention" (p. 255). Replication of the Epstein et al. (1990) findings are essential. Major funding from The National Institutes of Health (NIH) is needed to study the efficacy of various prevention and treatment programs in the prevention of childhood obesity. Such efforts could reverse the alarming trends in our youth toward a greater prevalence of obesity as early as 6 years of age (see chapter 7).

Genetic Aspects of Obesity

In studies on the genetic aspects of obesity, Bouchard (1989) points out several limitations of past research in estimating the hereditability of body fatness and the large range in conclusions in the literature, from studies indicating "little genetic effect" to studies supporting a "very high genetic effect" for obesity. In over 35 such studies using parents and their biological children, parents and their adopted children, brothers and sisters, siblings by adoption, and twin studies, two limitations are evident: (a) the genetic-by-environmental interaction and, (b) culture (nongenetic inheritance). Using some of the more recent tools of the genetic epidemiology, Bouchard, Pérusse, Leblanc, Tremblay, and Thèriault (1988) found that the additive genetic effect for body fatness was between 5% and 25%, depending on the body composition method used (BMI, sum of skinfolds, underwater weighing). The cultural effect was between 30% and 35%, and the nontransmissible effects (lifestyle, environmental, etc.) were 45% to 65%.

Recommendations Based on Tracking

So, what do we tell children at 2 years, 8 years, or 14 years of age, if we find them above the 85th or 95th percentile for skinfolds? Based on the literature reviewed in this chapter and the revised estimates of body composition of prepubescent children, we know that if 2-year-olds' skinfolds are between the 85th and 95th percentile (Johnson et al., 1981), they are probably less than 25% fat for boys and 32% fat for girls and that they are much more likely not to become obese than to become obese (Table 8.1). However, for those of these 2-year-olds whose parents (one or both) are obese and who are above the 95th percentile for skinfolds, I would predict a higher degree of tracking than that found by Garn et al. (1985), given some genetic and situational contributors. Pediatricians need to follow these children over the next 5 years and work with their parents to decrease the extent of obesity. Research, however, is lacking on this point and needs to be conducted in this age group of young children with parental obesity present. Eight-year-olds above the 85th percentile for skinfolds also will not necessarily become obese as adults, yet it is more likely than for 2-year-olds (Table 8.1). Educational programs are needed for these children, to insure a greater physical activity level and dietary evaluation, so that as they grow into adolescents they are well informed of their body composition and its potential modification with puberty and behavioral changes. For 8-year-olds above the 95th percentile for skinfolds, an intervention program is needed, and some combination of nutritional, exercise, and behavioral management is recommended. In addition, some children may need personal counseling to deal with their emotional development and self- and body image, which may be affecting their attitudes toward weight reduction and success in moving toward a more ideal weight. Finally, 14-year-olds at the 85th and 95th percentiles need an intervention program to help them lose weight and deal with the various nutritional, activity, and behavioral aspects related to their individual situations.

Table 8.1   Percent Fat at 85th and 95th Percentiles from NCHS Data

Variable	2-year-olds		8-year-olds		14-year-olds	
	85th	95th	85th	95th	85th	95th
Tricep and subscapular						
Male	19.5	25.0	18.0	25.0	29.5	42.5
Female	21.5	25.0	29.5	42.0	43.0	61.0
% Fat of sum of skinfolds						
Male	19	24	18	24	22	28
Female	18	22	17	33	33	42

Note. Calculations were derived using Johnson et al. (1981) data and Slaughter et al. (1988) equations.

Summary

The major focus of this chapter has been on the degree of tracking of body fatness from infancy to adulthood. Evidence was reviewed to indicate that obesity tracks best after puberty, and the level of fatness in infancy and childhood is not predictive of adult fat levels to any large extent. Children at higher levels of fatness do track to a greater extent than those at lower fatness levels in relation to adult obesity, and children from obese biological parents may also track to a greater extent. Estimates of the genetic effects of obesity have been recently modified, after accounting for the cultural effect, and range from 5% to 25%, depending on the method of assessment. Yet twins reared apart are much more alike in body mass index than expected (Stunkard et al., 1990). Additional research is needed using the more recent tools of genetic epidemiology and various methods of estimating fatness and fat distribution to resolve the issue.

Chapter 9

Body Composition and Youth Fitness

Assessing body composition using the skinfold method is part of a major effort in the profession of physical education to improve the health and well-being of youth. There is a shift away from performance fitness to an emphasis on the importance of a lifelong active lifestyle for prevention of various chronic diseases. Whether we can use skinfolds to give accurate body composition information to each child, while building self-esteem and healthy attitudes in youth, leading to a decrease in adult obesity, is now being tested.

Educating students about the relation of health to fitness and physical activity has been an important area for the physical education profession over the past 15 years. The American Association for Health, Physical Education, Recreation and Dance (AAHPERD) has provided leadership in the development of youth fitness tests since the first such test was published in 1961. In more recent years the Aerobic Institute has given health-related fitness much emphasis and direction throughout the nation.

Historical Perspectives in Health-Related Fitness

From 1975 to 1980 various committees dealt with the issue of performance-related fitness, which had been a major emphasis of youth fitness tests, and the need to emphasize health-related fitness. A consensus was reached that physical inactivity was an important contributor to three major diseases in the U.S. adult population—obesity, cardiovascular disease, and lower back pain—and that there was a need to teach children about the health benefits of an active lifestyle. The Health-Related Physical Fitness Test, introduced by AAHPERD in 1981, includes four test items: skinfolds to assess body composition, mile- run time to assess cardiorespiratory endurance, sit-and-reach test to assess flexibility, and sit-ups to assess abdominal muscle strength. The latter two tests are designed to help children learn about prevention of lower back pain, and the former two relate to the prevention of obesity and cardiovascular diseases. If children could learn to maintain their body fatness in an optimal range for health and increase their cardiorespiratory endurance, they would have acquired important knowledge for the prevention of these major diseases in the U.S. population.

At first, for the four tests, percentiles were used from national probability or convenience samples, depending on the item, to define age norms for female and male children. For skinfolds, children were encouraged to maintain their body weight if their skinfolds were above the 75th percentile and to lose weight if their sum of two skinfolds (triceps plus subscapular) was over the 90th percentile. With the development of the body-fat skinfold equations as explained in chapter 6 (Slaughter et al., 1988; Lohman, 1986), skinfold percent-fat charts were developed and published for the physical educator (Lohman, 1987) and presented at workshops over the next 3 years. These charts have now been adapted in prominent health-related fitness tests—Fit Youth Today (Texas), YMCA Youth Fitness Test, Fitnessgram (Aerobic Institute, Prudential), and Physical Best (AAHPERD; McSwegin, Pemberton, Petray, & Going, 1989)—to help children interpret their scores. Along with the development of percent-fat charts came the concept of using criterion-referenced standards for all four tests rather than norm-referenced standard norms. This approach uses percent fat as it relates to risk of disease rather than to norms and teaches children the level of fatness at which they increase their risk of experiencing, as an adult, hypertension, diabetes, elevated blood lipid levels, and, thus, cardiovascular disease.

The Fitnessgram was the first health-related youth fitness test to set up this criterion-referenced system for all four tests, with an emphasis on children with low fitness scores being at risk and the need to develop individualized programs to increase physical activity levels. For example, one child may have excellent cardiovascular endurance and body composition but need to increase flexibility. Another may need to emphasize weight loss and a more active lifestyle because of his or her risk for adult obesity and low cardiorespiratory endurance.

Making Body Composition Assessment Practical

During the 1980s, many professionals tried to make the skinfold test easier to administer. The subscapular site was not easily measured in females without their undressing or wearing loose clothing, so research was done to compare the triceps and calf sites with the triceps and subscapular sites. Because similar results were found with these two approaches, when corrected for bone and water content in children and youth (Slaughter et al., 1988), charts and tables were developed for the triceps and calf sites (Lohman, 1987).

Research also determined that videotapes showing the skinfold training procedure are as effective as workshops (Shaw, 1986) and offer an effective way to standardize skinfolds so that all in our profession use the same procedure. From a grant I obtained from Canyon Ranch of Tucson, Arizona, I made a videotape on measuring skinfolds on the triceps, subscapular, and calf sites and showed how to measure and interpret the skinfold results on children. Then I tested it out on over 100 graduate students ranging in experience from never having measured skinfolds to having considerable training and compared the results with results from a manual and from a workshop. From these findings I revised the audiovisual tape with the support of Human Kinetics Publishers, and for the past 3 years these tapes have been purchased by many professionals throughout the country.

The third development was to test various plastic calipers available from various suppliers (Appendix 9.1) to see if they compared favorably with the Lange skinfold caliper and Harpenden skinfold caliper (Figure 9.1). Figure 9.2 is a qualitative summary of the results of various tests, indicating that a plastic

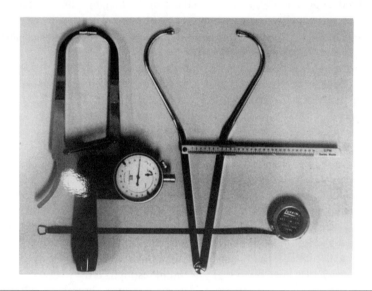

Figure 9.1   Harpenden skinfold caliper (left), anthropometric for skeletal widths (center), and metal tape for circumferences (right). *Note*. Photo courtesy of Timothy Lohman.

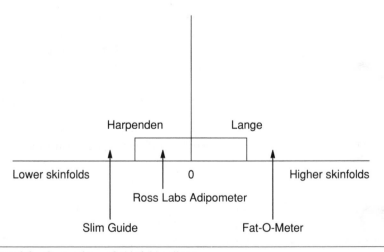

Figure 9.2   Comparison of skinfold calipers.

caliper can be used in place of the more expensive Lange caliper from which the national norms were developed. It has been found that even two excellent calipers, Harpenden and Lange, can differ by 1 to 4 mm, with the Harpenden giving lower values than the Lange (Lohman, Pollock, et al., 1984). A Ross Laboratories caliper gives slightly lower skinfolds than the Lange.

I recommend the Ross Laboratories caliper if the Lange or the Lafayette caliper (which produces results comparable to those of the Lange) cannot be purchased. The strong spring of the Slim Guide produces differential pressure as fat thickness increases and the weak spring of the Fat-O-Meter leads to higher skinfold measurements (Lohman & Pollock, 1981).

To make the interpretation of skinfolds easier I have developed computer software that can be used to produce a report for each child once her or his two skinfolds have been measured (see appendix 6.1).

Body Composition Testing in Public Schools

A model program of how this fitness testing works in the public schools is described by Sandy Blazer in the Going and Lohman (1990) response to a critique of skinfold tests by Riley (1990). In his response to the Going and Lohman article (1990), Riley (1991) states: "It is an erroneous inferential leap to assume that because a relationship exists between body fat and debilitative diseases that scientifically confirm such body fat and communicating the information to children will produce positive results and lower the incidence of childhood obesity" (p. 7). He goes on to say; "Skinfold testing is a relatively unimportant factor in alleviating the multifaceted problem of obesity. Improving self-esteem, teaching about proper nutrition and exercise, teaching movement skills and promoting physical activity will reap far greater benefits" (p. 7). With the exception of the research study by Epstein et al. (1990) discussed in chapter 8, there is little data to show how effective any of our fitness tests and programs are at changing the fatness, fitness, and activity levels of our children. In our argument with Riley (Going & Lohman, 1990), we call on our profession to develop a variety of approaches to the prevention of obesity, using skinfolds or other well-established body composition assessment methods to assess the changes in body fatness over a 2- to 3-year period. Riley, on the other hand, would omit skinfold assessment from the public schools on the grounds that it takes too much supervision and too much time and presents political, emotional, and social problems that are best avoided by dropping the tests. Riley shifts from, "Blazer's program is a tribute to the fact that skinfold testing can be made workable" (Riley, 1991, p. 6) to "Is it worth it?" (p. 6). This is a question to be answered by our profession in the 1990s.

Recently, I did a survey to follow up on some of Riley's ideas on those physical educators who attended a workshop ($N = 104$ responses) on youth fitness in October 1990 at the Arizona AAHPERD annual meeting. Arizona, as a state, has been receptive to health-related fitness testing, because of the efforts of many professionals to teach this new approach to youth fitness. Thus, 63% of those attending the workshop reported using skinfolds, and of those 66 individuals, 94% believe that skinfolds can be administered to yield valid results in the public school setting. In contrast, 47% of the 38 individuals attending the workshop who do not use skinfolds feel that they are poorly administered and yield questionable results. Additional results shown in Table 9.1 indicate that there are several aspects that must be integrated into a successful program if skinfolds are to be used successfully by a school staff that is well versed in the method and its application to youth fitness.

In the San Diego public schools, attempts are being made to increase children's activity levels with Fitnessgram testing, including skinfolds as part of the overall program. Such research studies are important to resolving the present controversy. In the meantime, physical educators such as Riley who decide not to assess body composition in children are left with their beliefs, but without any body composition data to establish that their approach is working to prevent obesity.

Elements of a Model Body Composition Program

Model programs interpreting health-related fitness including body composition assessment need to be developed and tested for their effectiveness in the 1990s

Table 9.1   Results of a Survey of Professionals on Use of Skinfolds

Those using skinfolds ($N = 66$)	Those not using skinfolds ($N = 38$)
96% Are familiar with the health risks of obesity and feel skinfolds help educate children about body composition.	50% Skinfolds tests elicit concerns about student sensitivity and right to privacy.
91% Want to follow changes in body composition over time.	37% Unfamiliar with the skinfold method and have not been trained by a videotape workshop.
88% Skinfold testing is worth the time it takes to obtain good results.	37% Too time-consuming and causes supervision problems.
82% Skinfold testing is an essential part of teaching health lifestyles.	31% Would rather use height and weight.
74% Have seen videotapes or attended workshops on how to measure skinfolds.	31% The skinfold test is an emotional and political issue and should be avoided.
	21% Measuring fatness in children makes me feel uncomfortable because of my own feelings about fat levels in myself and others.
	10% Do not feel ownership in the development of health-related fitness tests.

Survey conducted at the AAHPERD annual meeting, October 1990, in Arizona.

in our public schools. Body composition assessment could include whole-body bioelectric impedance as well as skinfolds and be integrated into the science curriculum as well as into the physical education curriculum to help students understand how the body conducts and resists current and how this can indicate the leanness and fatness of the body. Children could all be measured once during elementary school in the science class, as well as by physical educators; this would help them realize the importance of the concepts being taught by the physical educator. Alternative programs using the school nurse to assess skinfolds in all children will allow subscapular as well as triceps and calf skinfolds to be measured and the fat patterning to be assessed as well. Recent results indicate that in addition to total body fatness, trunk fat should also be assessed as an independent risk factor, because of the association of cardiovascular disease and central body fatness (see chapters 5 and 7).

Supervising Body Composition Assessment

One way to solve the supervision problem is to teach children to assess their own skinfolds (calf, abdomen, and biceps) and have plastic calipers (from Ross Laboratories) distributed to students in teams of three. Alternating in the roles of recorder, measurer, and subject, each student gets a turn to measure and be measured, and at the same time the physical education teacher can circle around the class and measure each student for triceps, calf and/or subscapular. Children can enter their own data into a microcomputer using the software, shown in Appendix 6.1 and obtain immediate results on themselves. Chuck Corbin, at Arizona State University, has been studying this approach for the past for the past 2 years and has found that students can self-test their skinfolds at the calf, abdomen, and suprailiac.

Maintaining the Subject's Self-Esteem

Children need to deal with their feelings about their fatness levels, fitness levels, self- and body image, and physical inactivity. Curriculum approaches need to be developed and tested to help children access and process their own feelings so that they can remove impediments to their self-esteem in any of these areas. Research of this sort is being conducted by Dr. Jim Sallis at San Diego State University. Such discussions need to be a part of the elementary and middle school curriculum, in health class as well as PE, and are critical to children's physical education.

Promoting Good Nutrition

Nutritional factors and eating habits and disorders that lead to excess or minimal fatness need to be discussed by all children throughout elementary and secondary schools. Restricting calories while improving the nutritional quality of the diet is a key element of weight reduction in tandem with an increase in physical activity. With the development of reward systems, such as those used in Fitnessgram and Physical Best, to encourage physical activity and fitness development in children after school and on weekends, teachers have the opportunity to help children assess their physical activity levels and encourage them to be active each day with a wide variety of experiences and activities. These events will help children experience their bodies in new ways, get in touch with who they are, and improve their self-concept to enhance their physical development and health. It will help balance our efforts to educate children physically as well as mentally and to increase their body awareness as well as their intellectual development. Such effects lead to greater self-esteem and healthier body composition and avoid more extreme efforts to lose weight.

Providing Information About Weight Loss and Body Fatness

Some professionals, ranging from members of the President's Council on Physical Fitness to occasional elementary school teachers who believe some children may become anorexic when told they are overfat, fear that using skinfold measurements in our schools will cause some children to lose too much weight. Because of emotional and cultural judgments against obesity or excess body fatness, many children have been insulted or criticized for their body fat levels. This is an unfortunate aspect of the world that the child must learn to deal with effectively. From my perspective, children have the right to select the fat levels they desire without suffering others' ridicule or prejudice, and they need to be encouraged to know the health risks and benefits, as well as effects on physical performance, that go along with excess body fat. They need to be given all the best information on how to lose body fatness through nutrition and activity-based approaches and on the harms and ineffectiveness of other approaches (e.g., crash diets, physical inactivity, poor eating habits, lack of body awareness, distorted self- and body images, fear of changing body type).

Tracking Body Fatness

The first aspect of a model program is developing a system to track changes in body composition such as that developed by the Utah Governors Council for Health, Physical Education and Sport. Such a system allows a child to follow his or her body composition throughout childhood and adolescence and gives important indicators to a teacher for excessive weight gain or loss during a given year of a child's life. Such an approach can help teachers intervene early with children who start to develop excessive leanness. With skinfold assessment each year, we may be able to become aware of a potential problem and, as in the case of the development of an eating disorder, refer the child to a school counselor for additional help.

Summary

Overall, the development of a model program to assess body composition in children has many elements, including psychological and nutritional aspects as well as an assessment of physical activity and body composition. Model programs may also need to include the parents, as found by Epstein et al. (1990). Those overweight parents who participated in an 8-week program of weight loss along with their children were still overweight to the same extent 10 years later, but their children were overweight to a lesser extent. This is one of the few studies to show long-term effects of a weight loss program for children. Such approaches need to be tested for their short-term and long-term results if we are to truly discover the essential elements in an effective model program for proper body composition development in relation to health. The key question to be answered in the 1990s is not whether to assess body composition in school-age children, but what program will be effective in decreasing the incidence and prevalence of obesity in children.

APPENDIX 9.1

The following is a list of addresses for skinfold caliper suppliers.

Harpenden Skinfold Calipers

H.E. Morse Co.
455 Douglas Avenue
Holland, MI 49423
(616) 396-4604

British Indicators, Ltd.
Sutton Road
St. Albans, Herts., UK

Lange Skinfold Calipers

Cambridge Scientific Industries
P.O. Box 265
Cambridge, MD 21613
(800) 638-9566
(301) 228-5111

Pfister Import-Export, Inc.
450 Barell Avenue
Carlstadt, NJ 07072
(201) 939-4606

J.A. Preston Corp.
71 Fifth Avenue
New York, NY 10003

Owl Industries, Ltd.
177 Idema Road
Markham, Ontario L3R 1A9
Canada

Lafayette Skinfold Calipers

Lafayette Instrument Co.
P.O. Box 5729
Lafayette, IN 47903
(317) 423-1505

Fat Control Caliper

Fat Control, Inc.
P.O. Box 10117
Towson, MD 21204

Adipometer Skinfold Caliper

Ross Laboratories
625 Cleveland Avenue
Columbus, OH 43216

McGaw Skinfold Caliper

McGaw Laboratories
Division of American Hospital Supply
Irvine, CA 92714

Holtain/Tanner/Whitehouse
Skinfold Caliper

Holtain, Ltd.
Crosswell, Crymmych, Dyfed
Wales

Pfister Import-Export, Inc.
450 Barell Avenue
Carlstadt, NJ 07072
(201) 939-4606

Chapter 10

Estimating Minimal Weight and Percent Fat in Athletes

Are population-specific anthropometric equations accurate enough to give useful estimates of minimal weight in the athletic population? In particular, can minimal weight be predicted in the high school male wrestling population with existing equations so that a nationwide approach can be implemented to prevent the health risks of dehydration and food deprivation characteristic of this sport?

O ne of the most determined and successful efforts to develop anthropometric equations that apply to a specific population is in the area of estimating percent fat and minimal weight in the high school male wrestling population. Over the past 20 years investigators have been working with skinfolds, circumferences, and skeletal dimensions to find the optimal equation. Contributions by Tipton, Tcheng, Sinning, Behnke, Wilmore, Housh, Johnson, Thorland, and myself, and many others have led to the publication of a landmark study Thorland et al. (1991) evaluating the validity of numerous anthropometric equations for estimating minimal weight in high school wrestlers. This chapter explores the success story behind the development of equations that have been cross-validated and can now be used throughout the country in this sport. Use of these equations may prevent the practice of acute weight loss and dehydration so well documented by Tipton and Tcheng (1970) and Tipton and Oppliger (1984). In addition, I will explore the development status of equations for other athletic populations and the need for further studies to cross-validate existing equations.

The Concept of Minimal Weight

The concept of minimal weight is derived from the application of body composition assessment to athletic groups for which a loss of excess body fat is associated with increased performance. In wrestling, long-distance running, and gymnastics, athletes are often encouraged to lose fat to maintain a lighter body weight. In wrestling, an additional incentive to lose fat is to wrestle at a lower weight classification, where opponents may be fatter at the given body weight and thus have less muscle mass and presumably less strength than the leaner opponent. In addition, there are several lightweight classifications that are harder to fill in high school wrestlers because most youth are considerably heavier and would have to lose 10 to 30 lb to reach the lower weight classes.

Behnke (1965) proposed that there is an essential amount of fat necessary for health. He defined lean body mass as fat-free body mass plus essential fat (for males, between 2% and 3% of LBM is essential fat). Due to measurement error and the belief that male wrestlers should have some subcutaneous fat in addition to essential fat, 5% fat has become accepted as the minimal amount that all athletes should have for optimal performance and health and to prevent loss of lean body mass (American College of Sports Medicine, 1985). Thus, minimal weight for males has been defined as equal to fat-free body mass divided by 0.95. Essential to a more refined definition of minimal weight is research studying the effects of weight loss below 5% fat on critical physiological functions. The effects on protein nutritional status, hormone levels, and physical performance decrements are essential to document in future research. We also need to know the effects of weight loss on growth rate and adult bone, muscle, and fat development.

Several anthropometrical approaches have been used to estimate minimal weight. In particular, skeletal dimensions and circumferences and, more recently, skinfolds and body weight have been used to develop generalized equations for high school wrestlers. Both approaches will be reviewed in the following sections.

Using Skeletal Dimensions to Estimate Minimal Weight

Early work with anthropometric dimensions focused on the association of skeletal dimensions and lean body mass. The Behnke and Wilmore (1974) approach utilized eight skeletal widths and height and assumed a geometric relationship between lean body mass and body diameters. The Hall method (Hall, Cain, & Tipton, 1965) utilized multiple regression analysis relating estimates of optimal weight to chest depth, chest width, hip width, height, and thigh circumferences in children. The empirical equations were developed from thousands of children and youth in Illinois. Tipton applied the Hall equations to high school wrestlers and found they overpredicted minimal weight. He then developed equations to estimate minimal weight in high school wrestlers, collected data on state champions, assuming all were at a 5% fat content during the final state competition. The following equation was developed on this sample by Tcheng and Tipton (1973):

Minimal weight, kg = 2.05 *ht* (in.) + 3.65 *chest diam* (cm) + 3.51 *chest depth* (cm) + 1.91 *bitrochanter diam.* (cm) + 8.02 *left ankle diam.* (cm) − 282.18.

This equation predicted minimal weight with a SEE of 8.9 lb (4.0 kg). Minimal weight was not estimated from underwater weighing or some other criterion method, but was actually the body weight of finalists at the 1968 to 1971 Iowa state wrestling championships; all finalists were assumed to be at 5% body fatness and thus at minimal weight. When thigh circumference was added to the multiple regression equation, the SEE decreased to 5.1 lb (2.4 kg). However, the equation with thigh circumference was not recommended, as its use overpredicted minimal weight in subjects with higher skinfolds.

Sinning (1974), in a critical evaluation of the diameter approach as compared to skinfolds, used densitometry in 35 college wrestlers to predict minimal weight. He found that the Tcheng and Tipton equations using skeletal diameters predicted fat-free body with a SEE of 4.0 kg, a result remarkably similar to that found by Tcheng and Tipton (1973), who did not use densitometry. Similar results were found by Sinning (1974) using the Behnke approach (1959) of eight skeletal diameters and constants derived from other samples. Results showing larger SEEs for prediction of minimal weight from skeletal diameters were found in high school wrestlers (Housh, Johnson, Kenney, McDowell, & Hughes, 1989) and in my review article on anthropometric predictors of lean body mass in adult samples (Lohman, 1991). We can see the implications of these results (SEE = 4 kg or 9 lb) by looking at the 12-weight-class system used by many high schools and recommended by the National Federation of State High School Associations. From 98 lb to 145 lb, each weight class has a range of only 7 lb. Above 145 lb, classes have ranges from 10 lb to 18 lb. The average 7-lb range for a given classification is smaller than the SEE of 9 lb prediction. Thus, a person's actual minimal weight could be 9 lb heavier than predicted, and the predicted weight could span over three weight groups.

Sinning (1974) also showed in the same population of wrestlers that fat-free body mass could be predicted with a SEE between 2.1 kg and 2.9 kg using skinfolds (subscapular and abdominal) along with skeletal diameters. This contrast of a 4.0-kg versus a 2.1-kg SEE between approaches is very significant. If we square the error and divide the larger variance by the smaller, an F statistic (a statistical test for the difference between two variances) of 3.6 is obtained. Thus, we see that the residual variance from skeletal diameters is significantly larger ($p < .05$) than that from skinfolds, for a factor of 3.6, and thus it is clear from the work of Sinning (1974) that the skinfold approach yields a smaller prediction error than the use of skeletal widths in the college-age wrestling population. If an equation can be developed in the high school wrestling population with a SEE of 2 kg (4 lb) or less, then we can use this approach in the field to help coaches and students achieve more realistic weight loss goals.

Finding a Valid Skinfold Equation for High School Wrestlers

The search for a valid skinfold equation for use on the high school wrestling population is best illustrated by two recent cross-validation studies (Housh et al., 1990; Thorland et al., 1991). In the former study Housh et al. (1990), using a sample of 409 high school wrestlers in Nebraska, cross-validated 23 equations drawn from previous studies in youth and young male adults. From the results of this extensive statistical analysis, the authors found four equations using skinfold thickness to be successful with total errors in density units in the cross-validation sample of between 0.0077 and 0.0090 g/cc and two equations with both skinfolds and circumference yielding SEEs between 0.0081 and 0.0085 g/cc. The errors correspond to percent-fat errors of between 3.3% and 3.8%, corresponding to minimal-weight prediction errors of 2.2 kg to 2.6 kg, using a 63-kg wrestler with an 11.6 percent-fat content. Two equations utilizing only height and skeletal diameters yielded total errors of 5.5 kg and 6.1 kg in minimal weight, confirming earlier work of Sinning (1974) in this high school population. The authors conclude that no single equation can meet all cross-validation criteria; however, of the six equations with several excellent cross-validation characteristics, they recommend the quadratic equation using the sum of three skinfolds from the combined work of Sinning, Sloan, Lohman, and Boileau (Lohman, 1981).

In the second cross-validation study, Thorland et al. (1991) analyzed data collected from five universities (N = 806 high school wrestlers). The landmark study was designed by Tipton, Tcheng, Kelly, Johnson, Thorland, Housh, Oppliger, Bowers, and myself. The sample of high school wrestlers from Iowa, Nebraska, Illinois, Minnesota, and Ohio was measured for selected anthropometric dimensions and for body density. All procedures were carefully standardized across laboratories before the data were collected. Thorland et al. (1991) found the total errors ranged from 2.4 kg to 2.6 kg in the best equations (Lohman, 1981; Thorland, Johnson, Tharp, Housh, & Cisar, 1984; Katch & McArdle, 1973). Thorland et al. (1991) also evaluated six new equations and changed the intercepts of the existing four equations to further test their predictability. Finally, these authors cross-validated the equations within three age groups and three weight groups to test for their generalizability.

The Effect of Age on Minimal Weight Prediction

In my review article on body composition assessment in children (Lohman, 1986) I combined the work of various investigators on the density of the fat-free body in children and youth as a function of age. Thorland et al. (1991) used these estimates of the density of the fat-free body as a function of age and computed the fat-free body using modifications of the Siri equation for age, as compared to one equation for all ages. They found that one equation gave a lower total error than the age-adjusted formulas I published (Lohman, 1986) and reasoned that the nonathletic male population between 15 and 18 years of age may be less mature and have a lower fat-free body density than the athletic wrestling population. Yet in an analysis of the constant error in their results (Thorland et al., 1991), the error was correlated in the same direction with the ages of their subjects in the several estimates presented in Table 10.1. Thus, the predicted minimal weights using the Lohman equation (1981), for example, show an overestimation of the younger group by 0.73 kg (mean age = 15.3 years) and of the middle group (mean = 16.7 years) by 0.34 kg and an underestimation of the

Table 10.1   Adjustment for Age of the Lohman et al. (1981) Equation for Estimating Minimal Weight

Age	Adjustment in minimal weight, kg
15.0	−0.89
15.5	−0.69
16.0	−0.49
16.5	−0.28
17.0	−0.08
17.5	0.12
18.0	0.32

Note. Data calculated from Thorland, Tipton, Bowers, Housh, Johnson, Kelly, Lohman, Oppliger, and Tcheng (1991).
Adjustment in minimal weight = 0.406 (Age − 17.2 years)

oldest group (mean age = 17.8 years) by 0.29 kg. The following equation compensates for this effect: Adjustment in minimal wt = 0.406 (age of subject −17.2). The use of this adjustment will account, perhaps, for the small difference in chemical maturity in the high school wrestling population and reduce the error as a function of age.

Finalizing a Skinfold Equation for High School Wrestlers

The credit for the development of population-specific equations for minimal weights in the high school wrestling population belongs to no one individual but to the cooperative efforts of many scientists. Each of us had his own viewpoint, yet in this case we worked together utilizing the ideas and efforts of each contributor for the benefit of the profession. Rather than rush our efforts into publication in the early stage, we continued presentations from 1987 through 1990 at the American College of Sports Medicine while sample size and refinement of the analysis continued until the final publication was completed (Thorland et al., 1991).

We have now reached a critical point, where this approach is ready to be implemented state by state throughout the profession. Without the efforts of Charles Tipton to encourage the five-university study, from its beginning with our meeting in Urbana, Illinois, in 1983, the efforts of Jack Kelly and myself to standardize all anthropometric and body density measurements, the extensive cross-validation analysis by Bill Thorland and Tse-Kia Tcheng, and the individual efforts of Dick Bowers, Terry Housh, Glen Johnson, Bob Oppliger, and Fred Roby, this success story could not have happened. Wisconsin has begun such an effort and is in the second year of a plan to use this system statewide in high school wrestlers. With equations now being developed in black and Hispanic high school wrestlers (Roby, Kempema, Lohman, Williams, & Tipton, 1991), the population-specific equations will soon be ready for general use throughout the country.

Thorland et al. (1991) cautioned that at best, however, the typical estimate of fat-free body and minimal weight has an error of ± 2.4 kg (± 5.3 lb). Further reduction of error is found within specific age groups and body weight data to as low as 1.7 kg (3.7 lb) in the lightweight groups, using the better equations (Table 10.2). Part of this error, however, is associated not with the skinfold equations but with the error in estimating percent fat from body density in this population, due to individual variation in hydration status and bone mineral content. I estimate that one half of the error variance is associated with the variability in the density of the fat-free body and that the 1.7-kg, 2.3-kg, and 2.6-kg errors are overestimates of the actual error by a factor of the square root of 2, or 1.2, 1.6, and 1.9 kg, respectively, for the light-, middle-, and heavyweight groups (Table 10.2). Therefore, if careful measurement procedures are taught to all testers, the use of these equations will result in a practical and useful approach for minimal weight estimation. The successful implementation of these equations will depend on trained technicians doing all the measurements with Harpenden skinfold calipers. Thorland et al. (1991) suggest that because of the potential error in the use of these equations, the judgment of a physician should also be considered in establishing a minimal wrestling weight. From a scientific standpoint I disagree with this suggestion and feel that an individual may request to be remeasured if he contests the results, but that we should avoid adding an additional subjective element into the assignment of weight class.

Table 10.2   Standard Errors of Estimate From Cross-Validation of Five Equations Within Categories

	Standard errors of estimate, kg[a]		
Equation	Lightweight group $FFB_x = 48.7$ kg	Middleweight group $FFB_x = 57.9$ kg	Heavyweight group $FFB_x = 68.8$ kg
Lohman	1.76	2.27	2.76
Thorland, et al. (1984)	1.79	2.45	2.32
Katch and McArdle (1973)	1.76	2.26	2.90
D2–Thorland et al. (1991)	1.68	2.24	2.75
D4–Thorland et al. (1991)	1.67	2.34	2.38
SEE, $\overline{X}$ kg	1.73	2.31	2.62
% of FFB	3.6%	4.0%	3.8%

[a]Standard errors of estimate within weight group and pooled across three age groups (Thorland et al., 1991, Table 9).
Note. D2 and D4 are specific equations in Thorland et al., 1991.

Population-Specific Anthropometric Equations for Other Athletic Groups

We are on the verge of developing population-specific anthropometric equations such as those discussed in the previous section on high school wrestlers. The need is great to develop equations for populations of different ages, athletic groups, and ethnic groups for both females and males. These equations could also be used to develop optimal as well as minimal weight predictions for a given sport. At the present time there is much evidence that the equation I developed from the data of Sinning, Sloan, Lohman, and Boileau (Lohman, 1981) is applicable to the high school wrestling population as discussed previously in this section. If we change the intercept from 1.0982 to 1.1030 g/cc, we obtain an equation that would probably serve the college wrestling population as well, based on the work by Sinning (1974).

High school white male wrestling population:
$$D = 1.0982 - 0.000815 \ (\Sigma \ 3 \ sk) + 0.00000084 \ (\Sigma \ 3 \ sk).$$

College white male wrestling population:
$$D = 1.1030 - 0.000815 \ (\Sigma \ 3 \ sk) + 0.00000084 \ (\Sigma \ 3 \ sk)^2.$$

Further modification of this equation for Hispanic and black wrestlers at the high school and college level may be needed, because the variations in fat patterning across ethnic groups affects the skinfold-to-fat-content relationship, resulting in a different equation for skinfolds versus fatness (Roby et al., 1991). Presently efforts are being made around the country to develop these equations in other ethnic groups.

The estimation of minimal weight in the female population has been investigated to a lesser extent, and the cross-validation of various skinfold equations in female athletes is needed. The work of Sinning and Wilson (1984) in the female population and Sinning et al. (1985) in the male population stands out, with various anthropometric equations applied to the athletic population. They found that the equation of Jackson, Pollock, and Ward (1980) using the sum of four skinfolds predicted very close to the mean density in the athletic population and had a low SEE and a good standard deviation of prediction values. Thus in the female population, I would recommend use of the Jackson-Pollock equation as follows:

$$D = 1.0961 - 0.000695 \ (sum \ of \ four \ skinfolds—\text{triceps, abdomen,}$$
supraliac, thigh) $+ 0.0000011 \ (\Sigma \ 4 \ sk)^2 - 0.0000714 \ (age, \text{ years}).$

If we substitute the mean age into this equation ($\overline{X}$ age = 19.82 years), we obtain:

$$D = 1.0947 - 0.000695 \ (\Sigma \ 4 \ sk) + 0.0000011 \ (\Sigma \ 4 \ sk)^2.$$

In our work with female adult athletes we used a different set of four skinfolds to predict body density (Going et al., 1990).

$$D = 1.0846 - 0.00064 \ (\Sigma \ of \ triceps \ + \ subscapular \ + \ abdomen \ + \ calf).$$

From these two equations we can derive the following results for guidelines for minimal weight for female athletes (Table 10.3). The mean skinfold for the sum of four skinfolds in the Sinning et al. (1984) female athletic population using the Jackson and Pollock (1985) sites was 69.5 mm, the mean density was 1.052 g/cc and 20.1% fat. For Going et al. (1990), the mean density for the population of athletes was also 1.052 g/cc (20.1% fat), and the sum of four skinfolds was 50.3 mm. When the same four skinfolds (triceps + abdomen + suprailiac + thigh = 55.7 mm) of the Going et al. (1990) study were compared with the Sinning sample, the skinfolds total 14 mm less. Thus, we see that the use of the Going et al. (1990) equation yields somewhat higher percent fat (3%) for the same skinfold thickness.

Therefore at this time we can use skinfolds only as a guide to estimate minimal weight on the female athletic population. We have two problems to deal with before we can proceed with a nationwide recommendation. One is the development of equations on a mixed sample of female athletes from several laboratories and universities to insure a generalized equation unlike the results shown in Table 10.3 and Table 10.4, where we have investigator-specific results leading to a systematic error in estimation of minimal weight. A second problem is that we do not have a good estimate of level of fatness corresponding to minimal weight in the female population. Different minimal levels of fatness are suggested by different investigators for women for health as well as performance. It is my view that some women may perform better at a higher level of fatness (e.g., 14% vs. 11%), other women, in contrast, may perform better at 11% body fat but become amenorrheic at that level and lose over time a significant amount of their bone mineral content. Finally, some women may perform best at 17%

Table 10.3 Skinfolds Corresponding to 17%, 14%, and 11% Fat in the Female Adult Athletic Population

% Fat	Predicted density	Σ4sk (Jackson-Pollock)[a]	Σ4sk (Going)[b]
17	1.060	55	38
14	1.066	45	29
11	1.074	32	17

[a]Sum of four skinfolds (from Jackson and Pollock [1985] = tricep, abdomen, suprailiac, thigh)
[b]Sum of four skinfolds (from Going et al. [1990] = triceps, abdomen, subscapular, calf)

Table 10.4   Comparison of Two Athletic Samples With Similar Mean Fat Content (20%)

Skinfold	Mean Skinfolds (mm)	
	Sinning & Wilson (1984)	Going et al. (1990)
Triceps	15.1	13.2
Abdomen	14.7	14.6
Suprailiac	13.9	8.4
Thigh	25.8	19.5

fat or higher, rather than at 14% or 11%, especially in such sports as swimming, basketball, volleyball, golf, and tennis, where higher amounts of fatness may not be detrimental to performance and may allow a higher level of nutrient intake and more optimal nutritional status.

Thus, as a rough guideline, at this time for swimmers I would recommend a sum of skinfolds of 45 to 50 mm using the triceps, abdomen, suprailiac, and thigh (%fat = 16% to 18%) or a sum of 38 to 43 mm for the triceps, abdomen, subscapular, and calf. For cross-country runners, I would recommend 12% to 16% fat for most, but not all, athletes and a sum of triceps, abdomen, suprailiac, and thigh skinfolds of 40 to 45 mm, or a sum of triceps, subscapular, abdomen, and calf of 29 to 34 mm. Further, cross-validation studies employing large sample sizes and interlaboratory cooperation are essential at this time to obtain more definitive equations for estimation of minimal weight in the female high school and college population.

Summary

In this chapter I have presented an overview of a 20-year research effort for a population-specific regression equation that could be successfully applied to the high school male wrestling population. The search started with the use of skeletal dimensions and proceeded to explore all anthropometric dimensions, including skinfolds and circumferences. Over the past 10 years, extensive cross-validation studies have led to the successful application of several skinfold equations in the high school wrestling population in the predicting of minimal weight. The most recent cross-validation study, by Thorland et al. (1991), serves as a model for interinvestigator cooperation and implementation of all essential cross-validation procedures. The result now awaits implementation throughout the country to help guide weight loss practices and prevent dehydration in this growing, active population. A change in the weight class system in high school wrestling to help minimize weight loss practices is overdue. More classes for wrestlers at higher weights are an essential component of a new classification system.

Other equations for female and male athletic groups are also reviewed, and recommendations are made for estimation of minimal weight in adolescent and adult populations. Further research using large cross-validation samples and multicomponent models are needed to establish valid prediction equations in various athletic populations. The concept of minimal weight in males and females needs additional research. The percent-fat level associated with significant physiological and metabolic function, and with a decrease in health for both male and female athletes, needs extensive investigation.

Chapter 11

Advances in Body Composition Measurement

As methods for assessing total and regional body composition become more accurate at estimating fat, bone, and muscle content, and as the link between body composition and health is being more clearly established, a general demand for reliable and accurate methods of assessing body composition is increasing in many settings, including hospitals, sports medicine clinics, weight loss centers, and public schools. This demand is being filled by both commercial efforts based on sound research findings and commercial efforts that exploit the demand without research backing.

In this chapter I will briefly explore new developments in assessing regional body composition and in multifrequency electrical impedance for fluid volume shifts, as well as address the important role industry can play in providing practical methods for assessing body composition. The role of industry in developing the total body electrical conductivity approach versus the infrared reactance approach illustrates the contrasting roles industry is playing. I briefly address further research needs, including new methods for estimation of muscle mass, new multicomponent models, better systems for estimating body composition changes over time, continuing interinstitutional cooperation to develop generalized regression equations using large cross-validation studies, and evaluation of model programs for long-term changes in body composition.

At present, industry has a large role in developing comprehensive body composition systems for hospitals, schools, weight control centers, sports medicine clinics, fitness centers, athletics, and research centers in nutrition, human biology, exercise physiology, and geriatric medicine. Much cooperation between universities and industry is essential to properly guide this development to best serve all populations, settings, and individuals.

Regional Body Composition

The need for new systems to accurately measure regional body composition is well established, given the link between fat distribution and health in the adult population. Methods that offer such estimates along with measures of whole-body composition will be in greater demand than those that measure only whole-body composition. New developments in dual energy radiography (DER), total body electrical conductivity, and bioelectric impedance all offer the potential to yield valid estimates of regional body composition. Careful studies, however, are needed for validation of each of these approaches. Segmental and total body impedance measures conducted by Going et al. (1987) and by Baumgartner, Chumlea, and Roche (1989) have not been validated using CT or MRI (magnetic resonance imagery) to determine their accuracy. DER appears to be an excellent approach to determining regional composition, because it yields lean, bone, and fat estimates of the arms, legs, and trunk. However, here, too, we need validation studies that determine the prediction errors of this approach and whether it can be used to assess changes in regional composition over time, as well as in the individual at a given time. Because DER can be used to scan the abdomen area to determine the lean, bone, and fat content, this method along with anthropometry may also be able to determine not only total abdominal fat but also the intra-abdominal visceral fat, as proposed in chapter 5. If this new approach yields valid estimates as compared to CT or MRI assessment of the abdominal region, DER could offer a more definitive assessment of the intra-abdominal fat on the adult population and its association with chronic diseases. Total body electrical conductivity also offers the possibility of estimating regional as well as total body composition as the body is moved through an electromagnetic field. Such systems will give scientists additional approaches to the study of regional body composition beyond the limited use of CT and NMR (Seidell, Bakker, & van der Kooy, 1990).

With better accessible methods to assess regional body composition now in the testing stages, soon to follow will be a reassessment of the use of anthropometric dimensions to estimate regional composition. The somatogram, for example, uses series of skeletal and circumference measurements adjusted by size of the individual to yield estimates of bone and muscle distribution throughout the body (Behnke & Wilmore, 1974). We can also use this approach for the assessment of fat distribution in the body from a series of skinfold measures. Further development of the somatogram concept has been proposed by Katch, Behnke, and Katch (1987). They separate the shoulder, chest, arm, forearm, thigh, and calf circumferences as estimates of the muscular component from waist, abdomen, hips, wrist, knee, and ankle as estimates of the nonmuscular components. Further validation studies are needed to determine the accuracy and usefulness of this approach.

In our work with regional body composition using segmental bioelectric impedance of the arm, leg, and trunk, we found the trunk resistance index to significantly improve the prediction of fat-free body mass when used along with whole-body resistance and reactance measures in both male and female middle-aged (30 to 50 years) populations (Williams et al., 1989). For a given whole-body resistance we found that as trunk resistive index (trunk length^2/trunk resistance) increased, fat-free body increased in both populations. In another study of segmental impedance, Baumgartner, et al. (1988) have examined the ratio of reactance to resistance (phase angle of the arctan X_c/R) in the arms, legs, and trunk and found that the phase angle of the trunk was a significant contributor to the prediction of percent fat (densitometry) in addition to skinfolds, age, and body mass index. Further investigations are needed to clarify the significance of trunk resistance and to determine the relation of regional body composition to regional measures of bioelectric resistance.

Multifrequency Bioelectric Impedance

The use of multifrequency bioelectric impedance analyzers is now possible with the cooperation of industry. One such commercial model can now be purchased (Xitro Technologies), and other units may be developed in the future. By varying the current below and above 50 KHz, it is possible to evaluate two critical questions related to body composition assessment:

1. Is there a higher correlation between body composition and the resistance index of the body at frequencies other than 50 Kilohertz (KHz) or with more than one frequency?
2. Are lower frequency currents (5 to 10 KHz) more sensitive to change in body fluids and the size of the extracellular space than higher frequency currents (Van Loan & Mayclin, 1991)?

If it turns out that in both cases multifrequency bioelectric impedance analyzers enable more accurate assessment of body composition and can detect relatively small changes in extracellular water, then we may have an instrument that can be used to assess acute and chronic effects of exercise on fluid volumes as well as body composition. Such an instrument will be able to give us more information on the controversy of Mazess (1990), Schoeller and Kushner (1991), and Deurenberg et al. (1991) associated with measuring body composition changes over time.

The Role of Industry in Developing Body Composition Assessment Methods

The role of industry in developing body composition assessment instruments that are based on sound theoretical and well-engineered construction with precision parts is crucial to reliable body composition assessment. Important to the success of bioelectric impedance has been the careful construction of instruments that yield highly reproducible results in their measurement of resistance and reactance of the body. The output of a constant 50-KHz current and an accurate assessment of the resistance of the body to that current is essential. These results have been achieved by several companies that have carefully engineered quality instruments.

The role of Valhalla Scientific has been noteworthy in supporting two large interuniversity studies to develop valid prediction equations for young, middle-aged and elderly subjects. A summary of these equations is found in Appendix

11.1 for equations based on several populations. Additional equations are given on children and the athletic female sample from the work of Houtkooper, Going, et al. (1989) and Houtkooper, Lohman, et al. (1989). One example of an impedance instrument that was not well designed was found in the results by Graves et al. (1989), who used bioelectric impedance instruments from Valhalla Scientific (Model 1990-A), RJL Systems (Model BIA-101), Medi-Fitness (Model 1000), and Bioelectric Science (Model 200z). In correlating the resistance values among instruments, three of the four different impedance analyzers correlated .99 with each other, whereas one analyzer (Bioelectric Science) correlated .60 with the other analyzers and with significantly lower mean resistance values (Graves et al., 1989).

Total Body Electrical Conductivity

An alternative to bioelectric impedance is the measurement of total body electrical conductivity (TOBEC), where the body is surrounded by a coil electromagnetic field. The measurement is based on the change in the coil energy as the body passes through the field. The conductance and capacitance change relative to an empty coil is measured (Harrison & Van Itallie, 1982; Presta et al., 1983; Boileau, 1988; Harrison, 1987). One of the first studies using this new method in comparison with others found that percent fat could be predicted with SEE of 3.7%, as compared to SEEs ranging from 4.7% to 6.9% for other body composition methods. These SEEs are all quite large compared to other studies (Segal et al., 1985), and this result may partly reflect use of densitometry as the criterion method in a mixed sample of men and women between 17 and 59 years of age. Soon to follow were research studies by Van Loan and Mayclin (1987b), Van Loan, Segal, Bracca, Mayclin, and Van Itallie (1987), Presta, Casallo, Costa, Slonim, and Van Itallie (1987) Presta et al, (1983), Boileau (1988), Cochran et al. (1988), and Horswill et al. (1989). Over 50 abstracts and research papers have been published in this area, leading to a consensus that this new methodology is a practical and relatively accurate method of assessing body composition. The role of industry in cooperating with university investigators has been a model for testing new methods. However, few studies have compared TOBEC with bioelectric impedance, so it remains unclear how much prediction accuracy is gained by investing in the large electromagnetic instrument needed for TOBEC assessment of body composition. It is essential that data already collected at several research institutions be published on this critical question.

Infrared Reactance

In contrast to the role of industry in coordinating closely with researchers in the field of bioelectric impedance and total body electrical conductivity, body composition by infrared reactance has not been studied as well and has had less cooperation between industry and body composition investigators. The original work of Conway, Norris, and Bodwell (1984) assessed fat thickness by infrared reactance and skinfold thickness by caliper and ultrasonics. Percent fat from body water was used as the criterion method, using deuterium dilution. The results were analyzed for 53 adults, and percent fat was predicted with a SEE of 3.0% for infrared reactance, based on the mean of five fat sites with somewhat larger SEEs for skinfolds and for ultrasonics. Infrared reactance is based on a spectral analysis of the interactance signal, which is, in part, a function of the optical scattering properties of the sample, with the amount of fat, water, and protein affecting the shape of the spectrum. Because other laboratories have not yet replicated the original work of Conway et al. (1984) with the sophisticated equipment available to her, the validity of this approach to measuring fat thickness throughout the body as well as body composition has yet to be established. Recent investigations into the area have worked with commercial devices designed with less precision and accuracy for distinguishing between water, fat, and protein and have not verified the original hypotheses, namely, that infrared interactance can be used to measure fat thickness more accurately than skinfold calipers because it is an objective measurement and does not involve fat compression. Researchers need to first work with an infrared interactance system similar to that of the Conway et al. (1984) investigation to firmly establish its validity and its improvement over skinfold calipers. With the cooperation of industry, such work could be accomplished before simpler, less expensive devices are mass produced. However, the lack of research in the area was exploited by one company promoting this technique as a valid method. This approach may have led to misleading results for many individuals. However, properly researched, this approach may yield an additional method of estimating subcutaneous fat in addition to skinfolds and ultrasonics. Its advantage over skinfolds in assessing the subcutaneous fat thickness layer throughout the body is the measurement of fat thickness without skinfold compression, but studies conducted to date have not shown great promise with present technology (Houmard et al., 1991; Israel et al., 1989).

Future Research Needs

The following research topics are presented to encourage others to investigate them: the development of more direct methods to estimate muscle mass, the need to define reference bodies for all ages and for both genders, the need to standardize body composition methodolgies, the development of effective programs to promote long term body composition changes, the need for valid multicomponent approaches, and the development of more accurate methods to assess body composition changes. These topics need particular attention and have numerous possibilities for future study.

Muscle Mass Estimation

The estimation of muscle mass as distinct from fat-free body mass or lean body mass has suffered from the lack of valid new approaches (Figure 11.1). Two developments have occurred since the novel approach was put forward to use body potassium in conjunction with body water content to estimate muscle, muscle-free lean tissue, and fat (Anderson et al., 1963). One is the discovery of serum creatinine to estimate muscle mass, with evidence in human and dogs of an association between muscle mass and serum creatinine level (Schutte, Longhurst, Gaffney, Bastian, & Blomquist, 1981). The second is the work of Buskirk and Mendez (1984) and Lukaski, Mendez, Buskirk, and Cohn (1981) showing a closer relationship between 3-methyl histidine and muscle mass, as determined by total body nitrogen and potassium, than to fat-free body weight. Further research, comparing these methods with the estimation of fat-free soft tissue by dual energy radiography and new methods yet to be developed, are greatly needed in the areas of growth, aging, and exercise training studies.

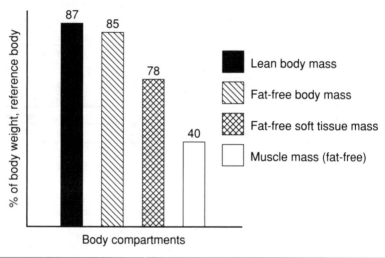

Figure 11.1   Percent of body weight of various reference components of the body in reference body.

Reference Body Composition

There is great need to extend the concept of reference body chemical composition to all ages and populations for both males and females. Although efforts have been made to characterize the change in chemical composition of the body in children and youth, much remains to be done to determine the effects of gender, age, physical activity, and ethnicity on the fat-free body (chapter 6). For example, Katch (1984) has hypothesized that body fat distribution in the reference female includes 5% sex-specific fat (breasts, genitals, subcutaneous, and intramuscular) and 4% essential fat (bone marrow, spinal cord, liver, heart, spleen, kidney, other) for a total of 9% fat for minimal weight in females. The muscle content of the body is given at 37% or a muscular content of 49% of the fat-free body. Continued development with multicomponent models will help to better resolve these estimates in various populations to establish reference bodies and composition, establish better estimates of minimal weight, and discover the links between minimal fat and health in both males and females.

New Multicomponent Approaches

The application of neutron activation analysis for the determination of several body components is one of the criterion methods available at Brookhaven National Laboratory and St. Luke's-Roosevelt Hospital, New York. Neutron activation analysis can be used to determine total body nitrogen using prompt gamma neutron activation, total body calcium, sodium and chloride by delayed gamma neutron activation analysis, total body carbon by inelastic scattering, along with dual energy absorptiometry, densitometry, and hydrometry (Heymsfield, Wang, Lichtman, et al., 1989). From this methodology Heymsfield, Wang, Lichtmann, et al. (1989) have developed several multicompartment models for the study of body fatness (Table 11.1). Because of the cooperation between Brookhaven and St. Lukes-Roosevelt laboratories, these investigators are in a unique position to develop and validate each of the four models for use in various populations and to make major contributions to the field of body composition in the coming decade that will enable us all to use simpler approaches more effectively.

Table 11.1   Body Composition Methods for Four Multicomponent Models Under Evaluation by Heymsfield et al. (1989)

	Body Composition Models		
1	2	3	4
Whole-body potassium	Total body carbon	Dual energy absorptiometry	Densitometry
Dual energy absorptiometry	Hydrometry		Hydrometry
Neutron activation analysis	Neutron activation analysis		Dual energy absorptiometry
Hydrometry	Dual energy absorptiometry		

Systems to Estimate Body Composition Changes

The estimation of body composition changes over time is one of the most difficult areas, because small-magnitude body composition changes are characteristic of many dietary and exercise-training variations. With changes in the order of 1% to 4% of body fat and fat-free body mass (Wilmore, 1983), it is difficult to accurately compare different treatment programs or know how to interpret the changes found (Lohman, 1986). In my review of selected studies using densitometry changes to compare running endurance programs with weight resistance programs, the mean density change in four studies for endurance training was 0.0040 g/cc as compared to 0.0030 g/cc for three weight-training studies (Lohman, 1986). Kushner et al. (1990) have successfully used bioelectric impedance to estimate body composition changes with dietary restriction, and Van Loan and Mayclin (1991) have used total body electrical conductivity to show body composition changes. Further research in this area includes the work of Ross, Leger, Martin, and Ray (1989) and Pennock (1990).

Future studies need to compare simultaneously several methodological approaches to the study of body composition changes, so that changes in other components of the body (e.g., water, mineral, and protein) can be separated from fat changes. Multicomponent models and new methodologies are needed to enhance our present approaches in this area. TOBEC, BIA, and DER all offer improved approaches for such studies and need to be used along with densitometry, hydrometry, and anthropometry.

Standardized Research Investigations

There is need for a national conference on the standardization of body composition methodology. Plans for such a conference for the fall of 1993 are under way under the leadership of Alex Roche, Elsworth, Buskirk, and myself. We plan to publish a manual from the proceedings similar to the Arlie Conference, which resulted in the *Anthropometric Standardization Reference Manual* (Lohman et al., 1988). By covering the major methods of assessing body composition we hope to reduce the methodological and procedural variation now characteristic of densitometry, hydrometry, dual energy radiography, bioelectric impedance, total body electrical conductivity, and other methods.

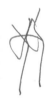

Along with such standardization we need to conduct research coordinated across laboratories with large data bases such as those by Segal et al. (1985) and Lohman et al. (1987), as described in chapter 4, and Thorland et al. (1991), presented in chapter 10. This cooperative research will help to guard against investigator-specific results and increase the generalizability of the findings. Such studies are essential if the national probability sample for NHANES III is to be utilized to the fullest extent with respect to total body and regional body composition data. From this national probability sample, we have the potential for the first time to develop body fatness norms for the U.S. population in relation to age, gender, and ethnic group. This will be achieved, I believe, toward the end of this century, leading to the general use of body composition standards in the U.S. population in all major health-related professions.

A Model Program for Promoting Positive Long-Term Changes in Body Composition

Once body composition changes can be accurately measured, there is a great need to develop model programs that effectively prevent obesity in children and youth and that help professionals deal with individuals who are seeking to reduce their body weight below their minimal weight for athletic or personal reasons. I predict that programs will be developed during this decade that will more effectively reduce the number of individuals with excessive fatness and yet decrease the prevalence of individuals below the minimal weight, where additional health problems can occur.

Summary

In this chapter I have presented some of the challenging new areas presently under investigation or in great need of investigation. I have also looked at the role of industry and body composition methods, indicating positive and negative contributions, with an emphasis on greater future cooperation between industry and universities because of the future demand in many professions for practical and accurate body composition methods. With the development in the 1990s of practical systems for assessment of fat, muscle, and bone, I expect body composition assessment to become a routine tool in the professions of medicine, physical education, and epidemiology, as it is now in the fields of exercise physiology, human biology, and nutrition.

APPENDIX 11.1

Bioelectric Impedance Equations Using a Valhalla Bioimpedance Analyzer

Population (age, years)	Regression Equation—FFB, kg					
	Ht^2/R	Wt	Xc	Intercept	N	SEE
Young adult females 18-30	0.476	0.295	—	5.49	153	2.1
Young adult males 18-30	0.485	0.338	—	5.32	153	2.9
Physically active females 18-35	0.577	0.208	—	6.73	47	2.1
	0.666	0.164	0.217	−8.78	47	1.7
Middle-aged females 30-50	0.493	0.141	—	11.59	121	2.5
	0.536	0.155	0.075	2.87	121	2.4
Middle-aged males 30-50	0.456	0.171	—	15.90	110	3.2
	0.549	0.163	0.092	4.51	110	3.0
Older aged females 50-70	0.474	0.180	—	7.3	74	2.8
	0.470	0.170	0.03	5.7	74	2.8
Older aged males 50-70	0.445	0.231	—	10.5	71	3.6
	0.600	0.186	0.226	−10.9	71	3.0
Male and female children 8-15	0.62	0.21	0.10	4.2	93	2.1

All *adult* equations can be corrected for the influence of FFB size on resistance by multiplying the constant .18 by the difference between the mean FFB in the sample reference and the predicted FFB for the subject. The sample reference means are: young adult females (18-30 years), 45.0 kg FFB; young adult males (18-30 years), 65.1 kg FFB; middle-aged adult males (30-50 years), 64.65 kg; middle-aged adult females (30-50 years), 45.3 kg; older adult females (50-70 years), 38.8 kg FFB; and older adult males (50-70 years), 58.9 kg FFB. This correction (mean FFB − predicted FFB) .18 is then added to the predicted FFB mass. All impedance is from right side of body.

References

Akers, R., & Buskirk, E.R. (1969). An underwater weighing system utilizing "force cube" transducers. *Journal of Applied Physiology*, **26**, 649-652.

Allen, T.H., Peng, M.T., Chen, K.P., Huang, T.F., Chang, C., & Fang, H.S. (1956). Prediction of total adiposity from skinfolds and the curvilinear relationship between external and internal adiposity. *Metabolism: Clinical and Experimental*, **5**, 346-352.

AAHPERD American Alliance for Health, Physical Education, Recreation and Dance. (1981). *Health related physical fitness manual*. Reston, VA: Author.

American College of Sports Medicine. (1985). *Position stand and opinion statements (1975-85)* (3rd ed.). Indianapolis, IN: Author.

Anderson, F.C. (1963). Three component body composition analysis based on potassium and water determination. *Annals of the New York Academy of Sciences*, **110**, 189-210.

Aristimuno, G.G., Foster, T.A., Voors, A.W., Srinivasan, S.R., & Berenson, G.S. (1984). Influence of persistent obesity in children on cardiovascular risk factors: The Bogalusa Heart Study. *Circulation*, **69**, 895-904.

Bakker, H.K., & Struikenkamp, R.S. (1977). Biological variability and lean body mass estimates. *Human Biology,* **49**, 187-202.

Baumgartner, R.N., Chumlea, W.C., & Roche, A.F. (1988). Bioelectric impedance phase angle and body composition. *American Journal of Clinical Nutrition*, **48**, 16-23.

Baumgartner, R.N., Chumlea, W.C., & Roche, A.F. (1989). Estimation of body composition from bioelectric impedance of body segments. *American Journal of Clinical Nutrition*, **50**, 221-226.

Baumgartner, R.N., Roche, A.F., Guo, S., Lohman, T., Boileau, R.A., & Slaughter, M.H. (1986). Adipose tissue distribution: The stability of principal components by sex, ethnicity, and maturation stage. *Human Biology*, **58**, 719-735.

Behnke, A.R. (1959). The estimation of lean body weight from skeletal measurement. *Human Biology*, **31**, 295-315.

Behnke, A.R. (1965). Discussion. In G.R. Menecky & S.M. Linde (Eds.), *Radioactivity in man*. Springfield, IL: Charles C Thomas.

Behnke, A.R., & Wilmore, J.H. (1974). *Evaluation and regulation of body build and composition*. Englewood Cliffs, NJ: Prentice Hall.

Berenson, G.S., McMahon, C.A., & Voors, A.W. (1980). *Cardiovascular risk factors in children: The early national history of atherosclerosis and essential hypertension*. New York: Oxford University Press.

Berenson, G.S., Webber, L.S., Srinivasan, S.R., Voors, A.W., Harska, D.W., & Dalferes, E.R. (1982). Biochemical and anthropometric determinants of serum β-and pre-β-lipoproteins in children: The Bogalusa Heart Study. *Arteriosclerosis*, **2**, 325-334.

Berkowitz, R.I., Agras, W.S., Korner, A.F., Kraemer, H.C., & Zeanah, C.H. (1985). Physical activity and adiposity: A longitudinal study from birth to childhood. *Journal of Pediatrics*, **106**, 734-738.

Boileau, R.A. (1988). *Utilization of total body electrical conductivity in determining body composition. Designing foods: Animal product options in the marketplace* (pp. 251-257). Washington, DC: National Research Council/ National Academy Press.

Boileau, R.A., Lohman, T.G. Slaughter, M.H., Ball, T.E., Going, S.B., & Hendrix, M.K. (1984). Hydration of the fat-free body in children during maturation. *Human Biology*, **56**, 651-666.

Boileau, R.A., Wilmore, J.H., Lohman, T.G., Slaughter, M.H., & Riner, W.F. (1981). Estimation of body density from skinfold thicknesses, body circumferences, and skeletal widths in boys aged 8 to 11 years: Comparison of two samples. *Human Biology*, **53**, 575-592.

Bouchard, C. (1989). Genetic factors in obesity. *Medical Clinics of North America*, **73**, 67-81.

Bouchard, C., Pérusse, L., Leblanc, C.,Tremblay, A., & Thèriault, G. (1988). Inheritance of the amount and distribution of human body fat. *International Journal of Obesity*, **12**, 205-215.

Bouchard, C., Tremblay, A., Deprès, J., Nadeau, A., Lupien, P.J., Theriault, G., Dussault, J., Moorjani, S., Pinault, S., & Fournier, G. (1990). The response to long-term overfeeding in identical twins. *New England Journal of Medicine*, **322**, 1477-1482.

Brozek, J., Grande, F., Anderson, J.T., & Kemp, A. (1963). Densitometric analysis of body composition: Revision of some quantitative assumptions. *Annals of the New York Academy of Sciences*, **110**, 113-140.

Bunt, J.C., Going, S.B., Lohman, T.G., Heinrich, C.H., Perry, C.D., & Pamenter, R.W. (1990). Variation on bone mineral content and estimated body fat in young adult females. *Medicine and Science in Sports and Exercise*, **22**, 564-569.

Bunt, J.C., Lohman, T.G., & Boileau, R.A. (1989). Impact of total body water fluctuation on estimating of body fat from body density. *Medicine and Science in Sports and Exercise,* **21**, 96-100.

Buskirk, E.R., & Mendez, J. (1984). Sport sciences and body composition analysis emphasis on cell and muscle mass. *Medicine and Science in Sports and Exercise*, **16**, 584-593.

Byrd, P.J., & Thomas, T.R. (1983). Hydrostatic weighing during different stages of the menstrual cycle. *Research Quarterly,* **54**, 296-298.

Chumlea, W.C., & Baumgartner, R.N. (1989). Status of anthropometry and body composition data in elderly subjects. *American Journal of Clinical Nutrition*, **50**, 1158-1166.

Clarys, J.P., Martin, A.D., & Drinkwater, D.T. (1984). Gross tissue weights in the human body by cadaver dissection. *Human Biology*, **56**, 459-473.

Cochran, W.J., Wong, W.W., Fiorotto, M.L., Sheng, H.-P., Lein, P., & Klish, W.J. (1988). Total body water estimated by measuring total body electrical conductivity. *American Journal of Clinical Nutrition*, **48**, 946-950.

Conway, J.M., Norris, K.-H., & Bodwell, C.E. (1984). A new approach for the estimation of body composition: Infrared interactance. *American Journal of Clinical Nutrition*, **40**, 1123-1130.

Davies, P.S.W., Jagger, S.E., & Reilly, J.J. (1990). A relationship between bioelectric impedance and total body water in young adults. *Annals of Human Biology*, **17**, 445-448.

Després, J.P., Moorjani, S., Lupien, P.J., Tremblay, A., Nadeau, A., & Bouchard, C. (1990). Regional distribution of body fat, plasma lipoproteins, and cardiovascular disease. *Arteriosclerosis*, **10**, 497-511.

Deurenberg, P., Weststrate, J.A., Hautvast, J.G.A.J., & van der Kooy, K. (1991). Is the bioelectrical-impedance method valid? *American Journal of Clinical Nutrition*, **53**, 179.

Deutsch, M.I., & Mueller, W.H. (1985). Androgyny in fat patterning is associated with obesity in adolescents and young adults. *Annals of Human Biology*, **12**, 275-286.

Dietz, W.H., & Gortmaker, S.L. (1984). Factors within the physical environment associated with childhood obesity. *American Journal of Clinical Nutrition*, **39**, 619-624.

Durnin, J.V.G.A., & Womersley, J. (1974). Body fat assessment from total body density and its estimation from skinfold thickness: Measurements on 481 men and women aged 16 to 72 years. *British Journal of Nutrition*, **32**, 77-97.

Enzi, G., Gasparo, M., Biondetti, P.R., Fiore, D., Semisa, M., & Zurlo, F. (1986). Subcutaneous and visceral fat distribution according to sex, age, and overweight, evaluated by computed tomography. *American Journal of Clinical Nutrition*, **44**, 739-746.

Epstein L.H., Valoski, A., Wing, R.R., & McCurly, J. (1990). Ten-year follow-up of behavioral family-based treatment for obese children. *Journal of the American Medical Association*, **264**, 2519-2524.

Foman, S.J., Haschke, F., Ziegler, E.E., & Nelson, S.E. (1982). Body composition of reference children from birth to age 10 years. *American Journal of Clinical Nutrition*, **35**, 1169-1175.

Forbes, G.B. (1987). *Human body composition*. New York: Springer-Verlag.

Forbes, G.B., & Amirhakimi, G.M. (1970). Skinfold thickness and body fat in children. *Human Biology*, **42**, 401-418.

Franks, B.D. (1989). *YMCA youth fitness test manual*. Champaign, IL: Human Kinetics.

Freedman, D.S., Shear, C.L., Burke, G.L., Webber, L.S., Harsha, D.W., & Berenson, G.S. (1987). Persistence of juvenile-onset obesity over eight years: The Bogalusa Heart Study. *American Journal of Public Health*, **77**, 588-592.

Frisancho, H.R., & Flegel, P.N. (1982). Advanced maturation associated with centripetal fat pattern. *Human Biology*, **54**, 717-727.

Garn, S.M. (1955). Relative fat patterning, an individual characteristic. *Human Biology*, **27**, 75-89.

Garn, S.M., & Lavelle, M. (1985). Two-decade follow-up of fatness in early childhood. *American Journal of Diseases of Children*, **139**, 181-185.

Garn, S.M., Leonard, W.R., & Hawthorne, V.M. (1986). Three limitations of the body mass index. *American Journal of Clinical Nutrition*, **44**, 996-997.

Garn, S.M., Sullivan, T.V., & Hawthorne, V.M. (1988a). Evidence against functional differences between "central" and "peripheral" fat. *American Journal of Clinical Nutrition*, **47**, 836-839.

Garn, S.M., Sullivan, T.V., & Hawthorne, V.M. (1988b). Reply to Mueller and Emerson. *American Journal of Clinical Nutrition*, **48**, 1343-1345.

Gluer, C.C., Steiger, P., Selvidge, R., Libesen-Kitcloth, K., Hayaski, C., & Genant, H.K. (1990). Comparative assessment of dual-photon absorptiometry and dual-energy radiography. *Radiology*, **174**, 223-228.

Going, S.B., Hewitt, M.J., Williams, D.P., Lohman, T.G., & Boileau, R.A. (in press). Estimation of total body water in older men and women by bioelectric impedance analysis. Manuscript submitted for publication.

Going, S.B., & Lohman, T.G. (1990). The skinfold test—a response. *Journal of Physical Education, Recreation and Dance*, **61**, 74-78.

Going, S.B., Lohman, T.G., Wilmore, J.H., Boileau, R.A., Van Loan, M., Sinning, W., Golding, L., & Carswell, C. (1987). Segmental versus whole body electrical impedance measurements for estimation of body composition. *Medicine and Science in Sports and Exercise*, **19**, S39 (abstract).

Going, S.B., Pamenter, R.W., Lohman, T.G., Carswell, C., Westfall, C.H., Perry, C.D., & Boyden, T.W. (1990). Estimation of total body composition by regional dual photon absorptiometry. *American Journal of Human Biology*, **2**, 703-710.

Gortmaker, S.L., Dietz, W.H., Sobol, A.M., & Wheler, C.A. (1987). Increasing pediatric obesity in the United States. *American Journal of Diseases in Children*, **141**, 535-540.

Graves, J.E., Pollock, M.L., Calvin, A.B., Van Loan, M.D., & Lohman, T.G. (1989). Comparison of different bioelectric impedance analyzers in the prediction of body composition. *American Journal of Human Biology*, **1**, 603-611.

Gray, D.S., Bray, G.A., Gemayel, N., & Kaplan, K. (1989). Effect of obesity on bioelectrical impedance. *American Journal of Clinical Nutrition*, **50**, 255-260.

Guo, S., Roche, A.F., & Houtkooper, L. (1989). Fat-free mass in children and young adults predicted from biotechnic impedance and anthropometric variables. *American Journal of Clinical Nutrition*, **50**, 435-443.

Hall, D.M., Cain, R.L., & Tipton, C.M. (1965). *Keeping fit: A 23-year study and evaluation of physical fitness tests* (pp. 1-38). Urbana, IL: Urbana Cooperative Extension Service.

Hangartner, T.N., & Johnston, C.C. (1990). Influence of fat on bone measurements with dual-energy absorptiometry. *Bone and Mineral*, **9**, 71-81.

Hansen, N.J., Lohman, T.G., Going, S.B., Hall, M.C., Pamenter, R.W., Bare, L.A., Boyden, T.W., & Houtkooper, L.B. (in press). Prediction of body composition in premenopausal females from dual energy X-ray absorptiometry. *Journal of Applied Physiology*.

Harrison, G.G. (1987). The measurement of total body electrical conductivity. *Human Biology*, **59**, 311-317.

Harrison, G.G., & Van Itallie, T.B. (1982). Estimation of body composition: A new approach based on electromagnetic principles. *American Journal of Clinical Nutrition*, **35**, 1176-1179.

Harsha, D.W., Frericho, R.R., & Berenson, G.S. (1978). Densitometry and anthropometry of blank and white children. *Human Biology*, **50**, 261-280.

Haschke, F. (1983a). Body composition of adolescent males. Part 1. Total body water in normal adolescent males. *Acta Paediatrica Scandinavica*, **307** (Suppl.), 1-12.

Haschke, F. (1983b). Body composition of adolescent males. Part 2. Body composition of male reference adolescents. *Acta Paediatrica Scandinavica*, **307** (Suppl.), 13-23.

Haschke, F., Foman, S.J., & Ziegler, E.E. (1981). Body composition of a nine-year-old reference body. *Pediatrics Research*, **15**, 847-849.

Hattori, K., Becque, M.D., Katch, V.L., Rocchini, A.P., Boileau, R.A., Slaughter, M.H., & Lohman, T.G. (1987). Fat patterning of adolescents. *Annals of Human Biology*, **14**, 23-28.

Heald, F.A., Hunt, E.E., Schwartz, R., Cook, C.D., Elliot, D., and Vajda, B. (1963). Measures of body fat and hydration in adolescent boys. *Pediatrics*, **31**, 226-239.

Healy, J.H., & Tanner, J.M. (1981). Size and shape in relation to growth and form. *Symposium of the Zoology Society of London*, **46**, 19-35.

Heymsfield, S.B., Smith, R., Aulet, M., Benson, B., Lichtman, S., Wang, J., & Pierson, R.N. (1990). Appendicular skeletal muscle mass measurement by dual-photon absorptiometry. *American Journal of Clinical Nutrition*, **52**, 214-218.

Heymsfield, S.B., Wang, J., Kehayias, J., Heshka, S., Lichtman, S., & Pierson, R.N., Jr. (1989). Chemical determination of human body density in vivo: relevance to hydrodensitometry. *American Journal of Clinical Nutrition*, **50**, 1282-1289.

Heymsfield, S.B., Wang, J., Kehayias, J., & Pierson, R.N. (1989). Dual photon absorptiometry. Comparison of bone mineral and soft tissue mass measurement in vivo with established methods. *American Journal of Clinical Nutrition*, **49**, 1283-1289.

Heymsfield, S.B., Wang, J., Lichtman, S., Kamen, Y., Kehayias, T., & Pierson, R.N. (1989). Body composiition in elderly subjects: A critical appraisal of clinical methodology. *American Journal of Clinical Nutrition*, **50**, 1167-1175.

Hines, J.H. (Ed.) (1991). *Anthropometric assessment of nutritional status*. New York: Wiley-Liss.

Hoerr, S.L., Nelson, R.A., Lohman, T.G., & Steiger, D. (1984). Relation of skinfolds to body fatness in a population of obese adolescent girls. *Medicine and Science in Sports and Exercise*, **16**, 135 (abstract).

Horswill, C.A., Geeseman, R., Boileau, R.A., Williams, B.T., Layman, D.K., & Massey, B.H. (1989). Total-body electrical conductivity (TOBEC): Relationship to estimates of muscle mass, fat-free weight, and lean body mass. *American Journal of Clinical Nutrition*, **49**, 593-598.

Houmard, J.A., Israel, R.G., McCammon, M.R., O'Brien, K.P., Omer, J., & Zamora, B.S. (1991). Validity of a near-infrared device for estimating body composition in a college football team. *Journal of Applied Sport Science Research*, **5**, 53-59.

Housh, T.J., Johnson, G.O., Kenney, K.B., McDowell, S.L., Hughes, R.A., Cisar, C.J., & Thorland, W.G. (1989). Validity of anthropometric estimations of body composition in high school wrestlers. *Research Quarterly for Exercise and Sport*, **60**, 239-245.

Houtkooper, L.B., Going, S.B., Westfall, C.H., & Lohman, T.G. (1989). Prediction of fat-free body corrected for bone mass from impedance and anthropometry in adult females. *Medicine and Science in Sports and Exercise*, **21**, S39 (abstract).

Houtkooper, L.B., Lohman, T.G., Going, S.B., & Hall, M.C. (1989). Validity of bioelectric impedance for body composition assessment in children. *Journal of Applied Physiology*, **66**, 814-821.

Israel, R.G., Houmard, J.A., O'Brien, K.F., McCammon, M.R., Zamora, B.S., & Eaton, A.W. (1989). Validity of a near-infrared spectrophotometry device for estimating human body composition. *Research Quarterly for Exercise and Sport*, **60**, 379-783.

Jackson, A.S., & Pollock, M.L. (1976). Factor analysis and multivariate scaling of anthropometric variables for the assessment of body composition. *Medicine and Science in Sport*, **8**, 196-203.

Jackson, A.S., & Pollock, M.L. (1978). Generalized equations for predicting body density of men. *British Journal of Nutrition*, **40**, 497-504.

Jackson, A.S., & Pollock, M.L. (1985). Practical assessment of body composition. *The Physician and Sportsmedicine*, **13**, 77-90.

Jackson, A.S., Pollock, M.L., Graves, E., & Mahar, M.T. (1988). Reliability and validity of bioelectrical impedance in determining body composition. *Journal of Applied Physiology*, **64**, 529-534.

Jackson, A.S., Pollock, M.L., & Ward, A. (1980). Generalized equations for predicting body density of women. *Medicine and Science in Sports and Exercise*, **12**, 175-182.

Johnson, C.L., Fulword, R., Abraham, S., & Brymer, J.D. (1981). *Basic data on anthropometric measurements and angular measurements of the hip and knee joint for selected age group 1-74 years of age, United States, 1971-75*. National Health Survey Series II, 219. Washington, DC: U.S. Department of Health and Human Services.

Katch, F.I., Behnke, A.R., & Katch, V.L. (1987). The ponderal somatogram evaluation of body size and shape from anthropometric girths and stature. *Human Biology*, **59**, 439-451.

Katch, F.I., & McArdle, W.D. (1973). Prediction of body density from simple anthropometric measurements in college-age men and women. *Human Biology*, **45**, 445-454.

Katch, V.L. (1984). A reaction to laboratory methodology. *Medicine and Science in Sports and Exercise*, **16**, 604-605.

Kramer, M.S., Barr, R.G., Leduc, D.G., Boisjoly, C., & Pless, L.B. (1985). Infant determinants of childhood weight and adiposity. *Journal of Pediatrics*, **107**, 104-107.

Kushner, R.F., Kunigk, A., Alspaugh, M., Andronis, P.T., Leitch, C.A., & Schoeller, D.A. (1990). Validation of bioelectric impedance analysis as a measurement of change on body composition in obesity. *American Journal of Clinical Nutrition*, **52**, 219-223.

Kushner, R.F., & Schoeller, D.A. (1986). Estimation of total body water by bioelectric impedance analysis. *American Journal of Clinical Nutrition*, **44**, 417-424.

Kvist, H., Chowchuny, B.,Grangard, B., Tylen, U., & Sjostrom, L. (1988). Total and visceral adipose-tissue volumes derived from measurements with computed tomography in adult men and women; predictive equations. *American Journal of Clinical Nutrition*, **48**, 1351-1361.

Lapidus, L., Bengtsson, C., Larsson, B., Pennert, K., Rybo, E., & Sjostrom, L. (1984). Distribution of adipose tissue and risk of cardiovascular disease and death: A 12-year follow-up of participants in the population study of women in Gothenburg, Sweden. *British Medical Journal*, **289**, 1257-1261.

Larsson, B., Svärdsudd, K., Welin, L., Wilhehnsen, L., Bjorntorp, P., & Tibblin, G. (1984). Abdominal adipose tissue distribution, obesity, and risk of cardiovascular disease and death: 13-year follow-up of participants in the study of men born in 1913. *British Medical Journal*, **288**, 1401-1404.

Lohman, T.G. (1981). Skinfolds and body density and their relationship to body fatness: A review. *Human Biology*, **53**, 181-225.

Lohman, T.G. (1982). Body composition methodology in sports medicine. *The Physician and Sportsmedicine*, **10**, 46-58.

Lohman, T.G. (1984). Research progress in validation of laboratory methods of assessing body composition. *Medicine and Science in Sports and Exercise*, **16**, 596-603.

Lohman, T.G. (1985). *Research relating to assessment of skeletal status.* Report of the Sixth Ross Conference on Medical Research. Ross Laboratories, Columbus, OH. pp. 38-41.

Lohman, T.G. (1986). Applicability of body composition techniques and constants for children and youth. In K.B. Pandolf (Ed.), *Exercise and sport sciences reviews* (Vol. 14, pp. 325-357.). New York: Macmillan.

Lohman, T.G. (1987a). *Body composition estimation for children* [computer software]. Champaign, IL: Human Kinetics.

Lohman, T.G. (1987b). *Measuring body fat using skinfolds* [Videotape]. Champaign, IL: Human Kinetics.

Lohman, T.G. (1987c). The use of skinfolds to estimate body fatness on children and youth. *Journal of Physical Education, Recreation and Dance, 58*, 98-102.

Lohman, T.G. (1989). Assessment of body composition in children. *Pediatric Exercise Sciences, 1*, 19-30.

Lohman, T.G. (1991). Antrhopometric assessment of fat-free body mass. In J.H. Himes (Ed.), *Anthropometric assessment of nutritional status* (pp. 173-183). New York: Wiley.

Lohman, T.G., Boileau, R.A., & Massey, B.H. (1975). Prediction of lean body weight in young boys from skinfold thickness and body weight. *Human Biology, 47*, 245-262.

Lohman, T.G., Boileau, R.A., & Slaughter, M.H. (1985). Body composition on children and youth. In R.A. Boileau (Ed.), *Advances in pediatric sport sciences* (pp. 29-57). Champaign, IL: Human Kinetics.

Lohman, T.G., Going, S.B., Golding, L., Wilmore, J.H., Sinning, W., Boileau, R.A., & Van Loan, M. (1987). Interlaboratory bioelectric resistance comparisons. *Medicine and Science in Sports and Exercise, 19*, S40 (abstract).

Lohman, T.G., Going, S.B., Hewitt, M.J., & Williams, D.P. (1990). Correlation of residual error with fat-free body and percent fat using bioelectric impedance equations. *Medicine and Science in Sports and Exercise, 22*, S109 (abstract).

Lohman, T.G. Going, S.B., Houtkooper, L.B., Williams, D., Pate, R.R., & Ross, J.G. (in press). Changes in skinfold and body mass index in children and youth over a twenty-year period. Manuscript submitted for publication.

Lohman, T.G., Going, S.B., Slaughter, M.H., & Boileau, R.A. (1989). Concept of chemical immaturity in body composition estimates: Implications for estimating the prevalence of obesity in childhood and youth. *American Journal of Human Biology, 1*, 201-204.

Lohman, T.G., & Pollock, M. (1981). Which calipers? How much training? *Journal of Physical Education and Recreation, 10*, 46-58.

Lohman, T.G., Pollock, M.L., Slaughter, M.H., Brandon, J., & Boileau, R.A. (1984). Methodological factors and the prediction of body fat in female athletes. *Medicine and Science in Sports and Exercise, 16*, 182-187.

Lohman, T.G., Roche, A.F., & Martorell, R. (Eds.) (1988). *Anthropometric standardization reference manual.* Champaign, IL: Human Kinetics.

Lohman, T.G., Roche, A.F., & Martorell, R. (Eds.) (1991). *Anthropometric standardization reference manual* (abridged ed.) Champaign, IL: Human Kinetics.

Lohman, T.G., Slaughter, M.H., Boileau, R.A., Bunt, J.C., & Lussier, L. (1984). Bone mineral content measurements and their relation to body density in children, youth, and adults. *Human Biology, 56*, 677-679.

Lohman, T.G., Slaughter, M.H., Selinger, A., & Boileau, R.A. (1978). Relationship of body composition to somatotype in college age men. *Annals of Human Biology, 5*, 147-157.

Lukaski, H.C. (1987). Methods for the assessment of human body composition: Traditional and new. *American Journal of Clinical Nutrition, 46*, 437-456.

Lukaski, H.C., Bolonchuk, W.W., Hall, C.B., & Siders, W.A. (1986). Validation of tetrapolar bioelectrical impedance method to assess human body composition. *Journal of Applied Physiology*, **60**, 1327-1332.

Lukaski, H.C., Mendez, J., Buskirk, E.R., & Cohn, S.H. (1981). Relationship between endogenous 3-methylhistidine excretion and body composition. *American Journal of Physiology*, **240**, E302-E307.

Lussier, L., & Buskirk, E.R. (1977). Effects of an endurance training regimen on assessment of work capacity in prepubescent children. *Annals of the New York Academy of Sciences*, **30**, 734-747.

Martin, A.D., Drinkwater, B.T., Clarys, J.P., & Ross, W.D. (1986). The inconstancy of the fat-free mass: A reappraisal with applications for densitometry. In T.J. Reilly (Ed.), *Kinanthropometry III. Proceedings of the VIII Commonwealth and International Conference on Sport, Physical Education, Dance, Rereation and Health, London.* New York: Chapman & Hall.

Mayer, J. (1965). Genetic factors in human obesity. *Annals of the New York Academy of Sciences*, **131**, 412-421.

Mazess, R.B. (1990). Do bioimpedance changes reflect weight, not composition? *American Journal of Clinical Nutrition*, **53**, 178-179.

Mazess, R.B., Barden, H.S., Bisek, J.P., & Hansen, J. (1990). Dual-energy X-ray absorptiometry for total-body and regional bone-mineral and soft-tissue composition. *American Journal of Clinical Nutrition*, **51**, 1106-1112.

Mazess, R.B., & Cameron J.R. (1971). Skeletal growth in school children: Maturation and bone mass. *American Journal of Physical Anthropometry*, **35**, 399-408.

Mazess, R.B., Peppler, W.W., Chestnut, C.H., Nelp, W.B., & Cohn, S.H. (1981). Total body bone mineral and lean body mass by dual photon absorptiometry. *Calcified Tissue International*, **33**, 361-363.

Mazess, R.B., Peppler, W.W., & Gibbons, M. (1984). Total body composition by dual-photon [153]Gd absorptiometry. *American Journal of Clinical Nutrition*, **40**, 834-839.

McLaren, D.S. (1987). Three limitations of the body mass index [Letter to the editor]. *American Journal of Clinical Nutrition*, **47**, 121.

McSwegin, P., Pemberton, C., Petray, C., Going, S. (1989). *Physical best: The AAHPERD guide to physical fitness education and assessment.* Reston, VA: American Alliance for Health, Physical Education, Recreation and Dance.

Metropolitan Life Insurance Company. (1983). Metropolitan height and weight tables. *Statistical Bulletin,* **64**, 2.

Moulton, C.R. (1923). Age and chemical development in mammals. *Journal of Biological Sciences*, **57**, 79-97.

Mueller, W.H., & Emerson, J.B. (1988). Functional differences between central and peripheral fat. *American Journal of Clinical Nutrition*, **48**, 1343-1345.

Mueller, W.H., & Wohlleb, J.C. (1981). Anatomical distribution of subcutaneous fat and its description by multivariate methods: How valid are principal components? *American Journal of Physical Anthropology*, **54**, 25-35.

Mukherjee, D., & Roche, A.F. (1984). The estimation of percent body fat and total body fat by maximum R^2 regression equations. *Human Biology*, **56**, 79-109.

National Health Examination Survey (NHES). (1973). *Sample design and estimation procedures for a national health examination survey of children* (National Center for Health Statistics Publication No. HRA 74-1005). Rockville, MD: Health Resources Administration.

National Children's Youth Fitness Study (NCYFS). (1985). *Summary of findings from National Children and Youth Fitness Study*. Washington, DC: Department of Health and Human Services.

Parízoková, J. (1961). Total body fat and skinfold thickness in children. *Metabolism*, **10**, 794-807.

Pennock, B.E. (1990). Sensitivity of bioelectric impedance to detect changes in human body composition [Letter]. *Journal of Applied Physiology*, **68**(5): 2246-2247.

Peppler, W.W., & Mazess, R.B. (1981). Total body mineral and lean body mass by dual photon absorptiometry. I. Theory and measurement procedure. *Calcified Tissue International*, **33**, 353-359.

Pierson, R.N., Wang, J., Heymsfield, S.B., Russell-Aulet, M., Mazariegos, M., Tierny, M., Smith, R., Thortnon, J.C., Kehayios, J., Weber, D.A., Dilmarvan, F.A. (1991). Measuring body fat: Calibrating the rules. Intermethod comparisons in 389 normal caucasian subjects. *American Journal of Physiology*, **261**, E103-E108.

Pollitzer, W.S., & Anderson, J.J.B. (1989). Ethnic and genetic differences in bone mass: A review with hereditary vs. environmental perspective. *American Journal of Clinical Nutrition*, **50**, 1244-1259.

Presta, E., Casallo, A.M., Costa, R., Slonim, A., & Van Itallie, T.B. (1987). Body composition in adolescents: Estimation by total body electrical conductivity. *Journal of Applied Physiology*, **63**, 937-941.

Presta, E., Wang, J., Harrison, G.G., Björntorp, P., Harker, W.H., & Van Itallie, T.B. (1983). Measurement of total body electrical conductivity: A new method for estimation of body composition. *American Journal of Clinical Nutrition*, **37**, 735-739.

Riley, J.H. (1990). A critique of skinfold tests from the public school level. *Journal of Physical Education, Recreation and Dance*, **61**, 71-73.

Riley, J.H. (1991). Skinfold testing—Riley replies. *Journal of Physical Education, Recreation and Dance*, **62**, 5-7.

Roby, F.B., Kempema, J.M., Lohman, T.G., Williams, D.P., & Tipton, C.M. (1991). Can the same equation be used to predict minimal wrestling weight in Hispanic and non-Hispanic wrestlers? *Medicine and Science in Sports and Exercise*, **23**, S29 (abstract).

Roche, A.F. (Ed.) (1985). *Body composition assessments in youth and adults. Report of 6th Ross Conference on Medical Research, Columbus, Ohio.* Ross Laboratories, Columbus, Ohio.

Ross, B., & Skoldborn, H. (1974). Dual photon absorptiometry in lumbar vertebrae: One theory and method. *Acta Radiology Therapy for Physics and Biology,* **13,** 266-280.

Ross, R., Leger, L., Martin, R., & Ray, R. (1989). Sensitivity of bioelectrical impedance to detect changes in human body composition. *Journal of Applied Phsyiology,* **67,** 1643-1648.

Schoeller, D. (1989). Changes in total body water with age. *American Journal of Clinical Nutrition,* **50,** 1176-1180.

Schoeller, D.A., & Jones, P.J.H. (1987). Measurement of total body water by isotope dilution: A unified approach to calculations. In K.J. Ellis, S. Yasamura, & W.D. Morgan (Eds.), *In Vivo Body Composition Studies* (pp. 131-137). London: Institute of Physical Sciences in Medicine.

Schoeller, D.A., & Kushner, R.F. (1991). Reply to R.B. Mazess and P. Deurenberg et al. *American Journal of Clinical Nutrition,* **53,** 180.

Schoeller, D.A., Kushner, R.F., Dietz, W.H., & Bandini, L. (1985). *Measurement of total body water: isotope dilution techniques.* Report of the Sixth Ross Conference on Medical Research. Ross Laboratories, Columbus, OH. pp. 24-29.

Schols, M.M.W.J., Wouters, E.F.M., Soeters, P.B., & Westerterp, K.R. (1991). Body composition by bioelectric impedance analysis compared with deuterium dilution and skinfold anthropometry in patients with chronic obstructive pulmonary disease. *American Journal of Clinical Nutrition,* **53,** 421-424.

Schutte, J.E., Longhurst, J.C., Gaffney, A., Bastian, B.C., & Blomquist, C.G. (1981). Total plasma creatinine: An accurate measure of total striated muscle mass. *Journal of Applied Physiology,* **51,** 762-766.

Segal, K., Gutin, B., Presta, E., Wang, J., & Van Itallie, T.B. (1985). Estimation of human body composition by electrical impedance methods: A comparative study. *Journal of Applied Physiology,* **58,** 1565-1571.

Segal, K.R., Van Loan, M., Fitzgerald, P.I., Hodgeson, J.A., Van Itallie, T.B. (1988). Lean body mass estimation by bioelectrical impedance analysis: A four-site cross-validation study. *American Journal of Clinical Nutrition,* **47,** 7-14.

Seidell, J.C., Bakker, C.J.G., & van der Kooy, K. (1990). Imaging techniques for measuring adipose-tissue distribution—a comparison between computed tomography and 1.5-T magnetic resonance. *American Journal of Clinical Nutrition,* **51,** 953-957.

Selinger, A. (1977). *The body as a three component system.* Unpublished doctoral dissertation, University of Illinois, Urbana.

Shaw, V.W. (1986). The accuracy of two training methods on skinfold assessment. *Research Quarterly for Exercise and Sport,* **57,** 85-90.

Sinning, W.E. (1974). Body composition assessment of college wrestlers. *Medicine and Science in Sports and Exercise,* **6,** 139-145.

Sinning, W.E., Dolny, D.E., Little, K.D., Cunningham, L.N., Racanielle, A., Siconolfi, S.F., & Sholes, J.L. (1985). Validity of "generalized" equations for body composition analysis in male athletes. *Medicine and Science in Sports and Exercise*, **17**, 124-130.

Sinning, W.E., & Wilson, J.R. (1984). Validation of "generalized" equations for body composition analysis in women athletes. *Research Quarterly for Exercise and Sport*, **55**, 153-160.

Siri, W.E. (1956). The gross composition of the body. In C.A. Tobias and J.H. Lawrence (Eds.), *Advances in biological and medical physics*. Vol. 4 (pp. 239-280). New York: Academic Press.

Siri, W.E. (1961). Body composition from fluid spaces and density: Analysis of methods. In J. Brozek, & A. Henschel (Eds.), *Techniques for measuring body composition* (pp. 223-224). Washington, DC: National Academy of Sciences.

Slaughter, M.H., & Lohman, T.G. (1980). An objective method for measurement of the musculo-skeletal size to characterize body physique with application to the athletic population. *Medicine and Science in Sports and Exercise*, **12**, 170-174.

Slaughter, M.H., Lohman, T.G., & Boileau, R.A. (1978). Relationship of anthropometric dimension to lean body mass in children. *Annals of Human Biology*, **5**, 469-482.

Slaughter, M.H., Lohman, T.G., Boileau, R.A., Horswill, C.A., Stillman, R.J., Van Loan, M.D., & Bemben, D.A. (1988). Skinfold equations for estimation of body fatness in children and youth. *Human Biology*, **60**, 709-723.

Slaughter, M.H., Lohman, T.G., Boileau, R.A., Stillman, R.J., Van Loan, M., Horswill, C.A., & Wilmore, J.H. (1984). Influence of maturation on relationship of skinfolds to body density: A cross-sectional study. *Human Biology*, **56**, 681-689.

Sloan, A.W. (1967). Estimation of body fat in young men. *Journal of Applied Physiology*, **23**, 311-315.

Smalley, K.J., Knerr, A.N., Kendrick, Z.V., Colliver, J.A., & Owen, O.E. (1990). Reassessment of body mass indices. *American Journal of Clinical Nutrition*, **52**, 405-408.

Smoak, C.G., Burke, G.L., Freedman, D.S., Webber, L.S., & Berenson, G.S. (1987). Relation of obesity to clustering of cardiovascular disease risk factors in children and young adults: The Bogalusa Heart Study. *American Journal of Epidemiology*, **125**, 364-372.

Stunkard, A.J., & Berkowitz, R.I. (1990). Treatment of obesity in children. *New England Journal of Medicine*, **264**, 2550-2551.

Stunkard, A.J., Jennifer, M.D., Harris, R., Pedersen, N.L., & McClearn, G.E. (1990). The body mass index of twins who have been reared apart. *New England Journal of Medicine*, **322**, 1483-1487.

Stunkard, A.J., Sorensen, T.I.A., Harris, C., Teasdale, T.W., Charkraborty, R., Schull, W.J., & Schulinger, F.S. (1986). An adoption study of human obesity. *New England Journal of Medicine*, **314**, 193-198.

Tcheng, T.K., & Tipton, C.M. (1973). Iowa wrestling study: Anthropometric measurements and the prediction of a "minimal" body weight for high school wrestlers. *Medicine and Science in Sports and Exercise*, **5**, 1-10.

Teran, J.C., Sparks, K.E., Quinn, L.M., Fernandez, B.S., Krey, S.H., & Steffee, W.P. (1991). Percent fat in obese white females predicted by anthropometric measurements. *American Journal of Clinical Nutrition*, **53**, 7-13.

Terry, R.B., Wood, P.D., Haskell, W.L., Stefanick, M.L., & Krauss, R.M. (1989). Regional adiposity patterns in relation to lipid, lipoprotein cholesterol, and lipoprotein subfraction mass in men. *Journal of Clinical Endocrinology and Metabolism*, **68**, 191-199.

Thorland, W.G., Johnson, G.O., Tharp, G.D., Housch, T.J., & Cisar, C.J. (1984). Estimation of body density in adolescent athletes. *Human Biology*, **36**, 439-448.

Thorland, W.G., Tipton, C.M., Lohman, T.G., Bowers, R.W., Housh, T.J., Johnson, G.O., Kelly, J.M., Oppliger, R.A., & Tcheng, T.K. (1991). Midwest wrestling study: Prediction of minimal weight for high school wrestlers. *Medicine and Science in Sports and Exercise*, **23**, 102-110.

Tipton, C.M., & Oppliger, R.A. (1984). The Iowa wrestling study: Lessons for physicians. *Iowa Medicine*, **74**, 381-385.

Tipton, C.M., & Tcheng, T.K. (1970). Iowa wrestling study: Weight loss in high school students. *Journal of the American Medical Association*, **214**, 1269-1274.

Van Loan, M.D., Boileau, R.A., Christ, C.B., Elmore, B., Lohman, T.G., Going, S.B., & Carswell, C. (1990). Association of bioelectric resistance impedance with fat-free mass and total body water estimates of body composition. *American Journal of Human Biology*, **2**, 219-226.

Van Loan, M., & Mayclin, P. (1987a). Bioelectric impedance analysis: Is it a reliable estimate of lean body mass and total body water? *Human Biology*, **59**, 229-309.

Van Loan, M., & Mayclin, P. (1987b). A new TOBEC instrument and procedure for the assessment of body composition: Use of Fourier coefficients to predict lean body mass and total body water. *American Journal of Clinical Nutrition*, **45**, 131-137.

Van Loan, M.D., & Mayclin, P.L. (1991). Use of multi-frequency bioelectric impedance analysis for the estimation of extracellular fluid. *Medicine and Science in Sports and Exercise*, **23**, 571 (abstract).

Van Loan, M.D., Segal, K. Bracca, E.F., Mayclin, P., & Van Itallie, T.B. (1987). TOBEC methodology for body composition assessment: A cross validation study. *American Journal of Clinical Nutrition*, **46**, 9-12.

Voors, A.W., Harsha, D.W., Webber, L.S., Rachakishmamurtz, B., Srinivasan, S.R., & Berenson, G.S. (1982). Clustering of anthropometric parameters, glucose tolerance, and serum lipids in children with high and low β- and pre-β-lipoproteins in children: The Bogalusa Heart Study. *Arteriosclerosis*, **2**, 346-355.

Wang, J., Heymsfield, S.B., Aulet, M., Thornton, J.C., & Pierson, R.N. (1989). Body fat from body density: Underwater weighing vs. dual-photon absorptiometry. *American Journal of Physiology*, **256**, E829-E834.

Williams, D.P., Going, S.B., Hewitt, M.J., Lohman, T.G., Graves, J.E., Sinning, W.E., & Wilmore, J.H. (1989). The prediction of fat-free body mass from segmental impedance and anthropometry in middle-aged men and women. *Medicine and Science in Sports and Exercise*, **21**, S39 (abstract).

Williams, D.P., Going, S.B., Lohman, T.G., Harska, D.W., Srinivasan, S.R., Webber, L.S., & Berenson, M.D. (1992). Body fatness and risk for elevated blood pressure, total cholesterol and serum lipoprotein ratios in children and adolescents. *American Journal of Public Health*, **82**, 358-363.

Wilmore, J.H. (1969). A simplified method for determination of residual lung volumes. *Journal of Applied Physiology*, **27**, 96-100.

Wilmore, J.H. (1983). Body composition in sport and exercise: Direction for future research. *Medicine and Science in Sports and Exercise*, **15**, 21-31.

Wilmore, J.H., & McNamara, J.J. (1974). Prevalence of coronary disease risk factors in boys, 8 to 12 years of age. *Journal of Pediatrics*, **84**, 527-533.

Womersley, J., & Durnin, J.V.G.A. (1977). A comparison of the skinfold method with extent of overweight and various weight-height relationships in the assessment of obesity. *British Journal of Nutrition*, **38**, 271-284.

Young, C.M., Bogan, A.D., Roe, D.A., & Lutevak, L. (1968). Body composition of preadolescent and adolescent girls. IV. Body water and creatinine. *Journal of the American Diabetic Associatio*, **53**, 579-587.

About the Author

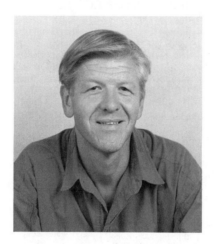

D r. Timothy Lohman is a leading scientist in the field of body composition assessment. He is a respected researcher, exploring both new body composition methodologies and body composition changes with growth and development, exercise, and aging.

Dr. Lohman is a professor in the Department of Exercise and Sport Sciences at the University of Arizona. He earned his PhD from the University of Illinois, where he was also a professor for 15 years. He is the author of many research articles and is one of the editors of the *Anthropometric Standardization Reference Manual*, published by Human Kinetics. Dr. Lohman also developed *Measuring Body Fat Using Skinfolds*, a Human Kinetics video that demonstrates how to measure body fat using skinfold calipers.

Dr. Lohman is a fellow of the American Academy of Physical Education, a member of the American College of Sports Medicine, a member of the youth fitness advisory committee of the Cooper Institute for Aerobics Research in Dallas, Texas, and a member of the Arizona Governor's Council of Health, Physical Fitness, and Sports. He serves as a reviewer for many scholarly publications, including *Medicine and Science in Sports and Exercise, Research Quarterly for Exercise and Sport,* and *The Physician and Sportsmedicine.*

Index